MW00377391

ESSENTIAL
KETO
DESSERTS

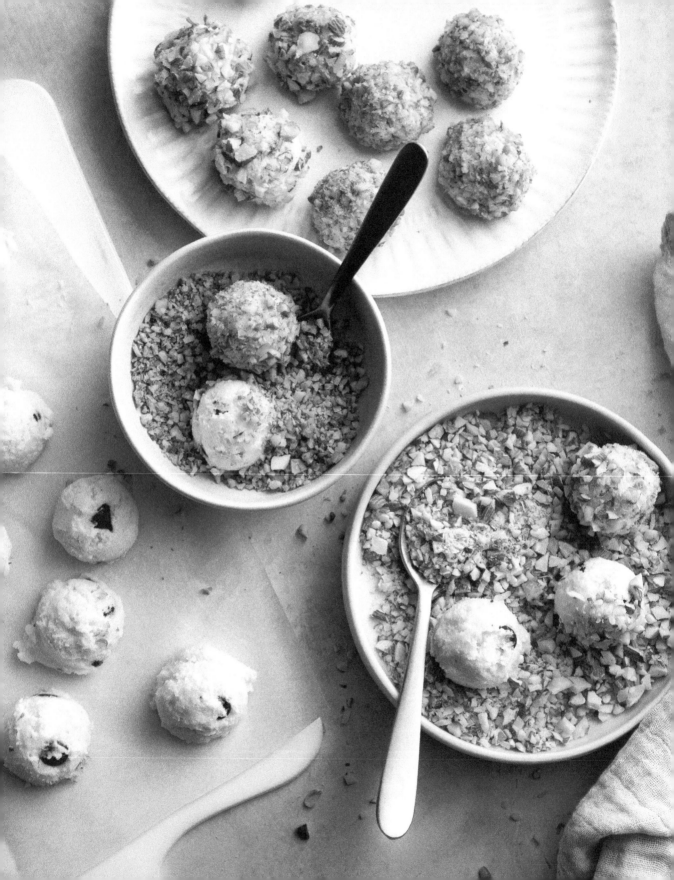

essential
KETO
DESSERTS

85 Delicious, Low-Carb Recipes to Satisfy Your Sweet Tooth

By Hilda Solares

Photography by Annie Martin

ROCKRIDGE
PRESS

Copyright © 2020 by Rockridge Press, Emeryville, California

No part of this publication may be reproduced, stored in a retrieval system, or transmitted in any form or by any means, electronic, mechanical, photocopying, recording, scanning, or otherwise, except as permitted under Sections 107 or 108 of the 1976 United States Copyright Act, without the prior written permission of the Publisher. Requests to the Publisher for permission should be addressed to the Permissions Department, Rockridge Press, 6005 Shellmound Street, Suite 175, Emeryville, CA 94608.

Limit of Liability/Disclaimer of Warranty: The Publisher and the author make no representations or warranties with respect to the accuracy or completeness of the contents of this work and specifically disclaim all warranties, including without limitation warranties of fitness for a particular purpose. No warranty may be created or extended by sales or promotional materials. The advice and strategies contained herein may not be suitable for every situation. This work is sold with the understanding that the Publisher is not engaged in rendering medical, legal, or other professional advice or services. If professional assistance is required, the services of a competent professional person should be sought. Neither the Publisher nor the author shall be liable for damages arising herefrom. The fact that an individual, organization, or website is referred to in this work as a citation and/or potential source of further information does not mean that the author or the Publisher endorses the information the individual, organization, or website may provide or recommendations they/it may make. Further, readers should be aware that websites listed in this work may have changed or disappeared between when this work was written and when it is read.

For general information on our other products and services or to obtain technical support, please contact our Customer Care Department within the United States at (866) 744-2665, or outside the United States at (510) 253-0500.

Rockridge Press publishes its books in a variety of electronic and print formats. Some content that appears in print may not be available in electronic books, and vice versa.

TRADEMARKS: Rockridge Press and the Rockridge Press logo are trademarks or registered trademarks of Callisto Media Inc. and/or its affiliates, in the United States and other countries, and may not be used without written permission. All other trademarks are the property of their respective owners. Rockridge Press is not associated with any product or vendor mentioned in this book.

Interior and Cover Designer: Jami Spittler
Art Producer: Sue Bischofberger
Editor: Ada Fung
Production Manager: Riley Hoffman
Production Editor: Melissa Edeburn

Photography © 2020 Annie Martin. Food styling by Oscar Molinar.

Cover: Raspberry Mousse Tart
Page ii photo: Cookie Dough Fat Bombs

ISBN: Print 978-1-64611-913-4
eBook 978-1-64611-914-1

R0

For my husband, Randy,
my champion.

For Michelle, Matthew, and Peter,
my children who gave me
the courage to believe.

ICED GINGERBREAD
COOKIES, P. 63

contents

Introduction ix

CHAPTER ONE
Living the Sweet Keto Life 1

CHAPTER TWO
Your Keto Dessert Kitchen 9

CHAPTER THREE
Candies, Confections,
and Fat Bombs 23

CHAPTER FOUR
Custards, Puddings,
and Mousses 39

CHAPTER FIVE
Cookies, Brownies,
and Bars 59

CHAPTER SIX
Cakes and Breads 87

CHAPTER SEVEN
Pies and Tarts 121

CHAPTER EIGHT
Drinks and Frozen Treats 143

CHAPTER NINE
Frostings, Toppings,
Sauces, Oh My! 159

Measurement Conversions 171

Resources 172

Index 174

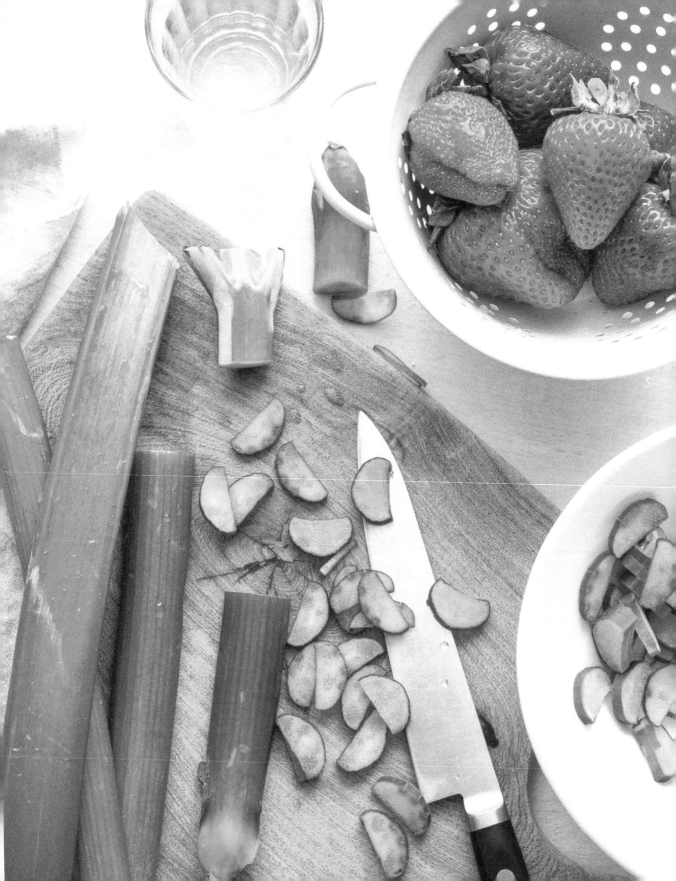

Introduction

I was diagnosed with Guillain-Barré syndrome and fibromyalgia in 2001. It felt like a life sentence of pain and weakness. Thankfully, this was not the case.

In 2006, after years of battling symptoms and only getting worse, I made the difficult decision to leave my life-long academic career. Uncertain of my future, I cried out to God for an answer. His response was simple: Remove sugar and grains from your diet. I obeyed, and it was then I inadvertently tapped into the benefits of the ketogenic diet.

For two years, I was committed to my diet, and my health dramatically improved. Unfortunately, my carb cravings got the best of me, and I returned to my old eating patterns. That decision caused my health to quickly spiral out of control. I ended up needing a walker, and was placed on a morphine patch for almost a year.

At the end of 2013, I saw the error of my ways and realized that abstaining from sugar and grains was the only way to get on the path to better health. So, in January 2014, both my husband, Randy, and I decided to make the keto way of eating a lifestyle. I became inspired to experiment and formulate sweet and savory keto-friendly dishes. Those first attempts in the kitchen were frustrating, but I was determined to make the lifestyle work this time around.

The transformation we experienced was dramatic. Randy lost more than 80 pounds and reversed his diabetes. I regained strength and got rid of the fatigue that had plagued me. We experienced these benefits because I was able to create recipes that helped us both stay committed.

When our family and friends saw the results, they wanted to learn what we were doing. Pastors Ricky and Yvette Gallinar gave us the green light to form a community group through which we have since supported others who want similar results. Our blog, FitToServeGroup.com, became our vehicle to share our journey, tips for others who want to go keto, and my low-carb keto recipes.

Having experienced keto's benefits firsthand, I am passionate about creating recipes that make the lifestyle more accessible. I wrote *Essential Keto Desserts* because I wanted to offer a resource for those with a sweet tooth. I hope this book helps you see the results you desire.

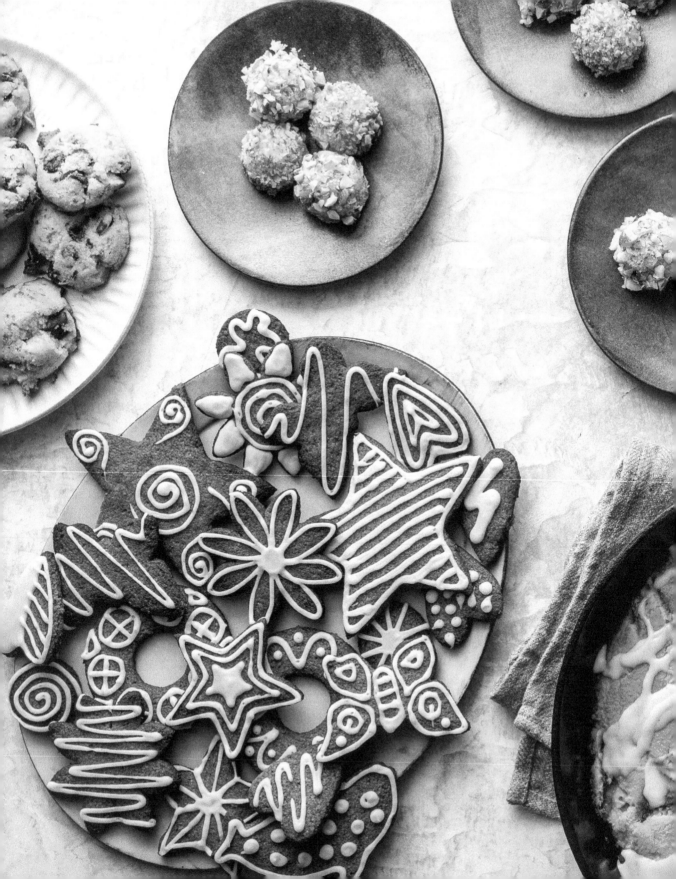

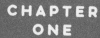

CHAPTER ONE

Living the Sweet Keto Life

When I first started keto, my constant cravings for sugary, high-carb desserts nearly caused me to give up. By creating my own keto dessert recipes, I was able to stay true to the diet—and have cake! In this chapter, I will show you how to do the same. I'll walk you through the basics of the keto diet, explain how to tailor your macros to include dessert, and give you some tips for making delicious keto sweets.

Why Have Your Dessert and Keto, Too?

One of the most challenging aspects of going keto is the prospect of leaving desserts behind. I get it; if there's anyone who understands the pull of sweets, it is undoubtedly me. But what if I told you there is no need to feel deprived? Having dessert while doing keto is not only possible but also encouraged as a way to stay committed.

Yes, you can have your dessert and keto, too! You can turn what was a weakness into a strength. My sweet tooth is the main reason I learned how to create keto-friendly desserts, which have ensured I stay the course and reap the long-term benefits of the keto diet.

With the right recipes, you, too, can curb the pull of carbs. *Essential Keto Desserts* is full of recipes for cookies, cakes, pies, mousses, frozen treats, beverages, and so much more. I am confident it will prove to be a valuable keto diet tool.

My "Natural Flavors First, Sweetener Second" Philosophy

The advent of keto-friendly sugar substitutes like erythritol, monk fruit, and stevia has allowed us keto-ers to enjoy desserts while adhering to the keto diet. However, these keto-friendly options have drawbacks. Erythritol, for example, can have an intensely cooling aftertaste and can cause bloating or other gut discomfort for some people when consumed in large quantities.

I also believe that part of the goal of the keto diet is to re-train our bodies to reduce carb and sugary food cravings. Consequently, I have a "natural flavors first" philosophy regarding keto desserts.

It's possible to create delicious and satiating desserts without depending just on sugar substitutes. This book's recipes aim to rely mainly on natural ingredients such as lemon and lime juice and zest, spices, extracts, berries, nut butters, cream, and cocoa powder for flavor. Wherever possible, I have included two levels of sweetener in the ingredients list, so you can tailor the sweetness of the dessert to your taste. As you become keto adapted, your carb and sugar cravings should naturally lessen, and you won't need as much sweetener to satisfy your sweet tooth!

A Quick Keto Review

The keto diet has gained a lot of popularity, and many have testified to its effectiveness in helping them lose weight, control cravings, improve cognition and energy levels, and even prevent or alleviate symptoms of chronic diseases.

If you're picking up a keto desserts book, I'm guessing you already have a working knowledge of the keto diet. For those who want it, here's a refresher.

What Is Keto and How Does It Work?

Our bodies are designed to be fueled by either glucose (sugar) or ketones (fat). The goal of the ketogenic diet is to transition your body into a state of therapeutic ketosis, in which you are burning fat rather than glucose. Ketosis is, essentially, the state of having elevated ketone levels of 0.5 millimoles per liter or more. How ketosis is achieved and how high blood ketone levels will be varies from individual to individual.

How does one get into ketosis? By eating a diet very low in carbohydrates, you essentially "starve" your body of glucose and eventually deplete the stored glycogen in your liver, which then forces your body to look for an alternative source of energy—dietary fat and stored fat. When fat is broken down by your body, ketones are released that your brain and other organs can then use for energy.

The fat-burning properties of ketosis are why so many people turn to the keto diet for fat loss. But there are other benefits to being in ketosis. Ketones are a more sustainable and continuous fuel source, which is why people on keto report feeling satiated for longer—they don't experience the periodic dipping that occurs when we are strictly glucose burners. Ketones are also the fuel source our brains seem to prefer, which is why people on the keto diet also report feeling more energized and focused.

You can determine if you are in ketosis in a number of ways such as by using urine strips, breath meters, and even blood tests via a finger prick. Many of these tests are available at your local pharmacy, whereas others, like the blood tests, are easier to source online.

Know Your Macros: Low Carb, Moderate Protein, High Fat

Success on the keto diet depends on managing your macronutrients, or macros: carbs, fat, and proteins. The diet consists of 50 grams or fewer of net carbs per day (net carbs are total carbs minus fiber). Only 5 to 10 percent of your total daily calories should come from carbohydrates. Keeping your carb intake low is important because you want to prevent spikes in blood glucose and insulin, which will stop your body from entering ketosis.

You want to keep your intake of protein moderate—somewhere between 15 and 30 percent of your daily calories. Eating more protein than this can make it harder for you to get into ketosis and stay there. If you're more active, you can likely be on the higher end of protein intake and still be in ketosis.

The main difference between a ketogenic diet and a general low-carb diet is the keto diet is high in fat. About 75 percent of your total daily calories should come from fat, but not just any fat—you want to include high-quality, natural forms of saturated and unsaturated fats like lard, butter, coconut oil, olive oil, and nut oils. You should avoid consuming trans fats, which are primarily found in processed and fast foods.

Everybody is different, and everybody's needs are different. To reap the benefits of the keto diet, you will have to personalize your macros to your own set of goals and unique circumstances. The good news is there are many free keto calculators online to assist you in determining your macros, such as the one on PerfectKeto.com. Once you figure out your personal macro numbers, you can plan your meals effectively—and figure out how to fit in dessert.

Fitting Desserts into Your Keto Lifestyle

How well you manage your fat, protein, and carbohydrate macros makes all the difference in how well you do on the keto diet. The recipes in this book are sugar-free and lower in carbs than traditional desserts. However, some of these recipes are on the higher end of the keto-approved carb count because it is challenging to make desserts extremely low in carbs. Generally, you will find fat bombs and mousses at the lower end of the carb spectrum, whereas layered cakes and cookies are more likely to be higher and should be an occasional treat, not an everyday item.

What is terrific about the keto diet is the flexibility it has for balancing your macros in a way that allows you to splurge on dessert. For example, if you want to have a treat after dinner, plan on having a smaller breakfast or lunch that day. By lowering your servings or changing an allocated meal for the day, you can enjoy dessert but still keep your daily macros in check.

The Deal with Keto Desserts

At first, the idea of making keto desserts can be intimidating because you will need to buy ingredients that may be completely new to you, and because there may be a learning curve for using those ingredients. Thankfully, you will be rewarded with the ability to have low-carb and nutrition-packed desserts. All the recipes included in this book use real whole foods such as butter and cream as well as nut flours and high-fiber options like coconut and flaxseed meal. These are superior to all-purpose white flour and white sugar, both of which equate to empty calories.

Although using gluten-free ingredients means having a different texture from a particular recipe's conventional counterparts, you can still achieve similar results. For instance, baked goods may be a little denser, and therefore require, say, more baking powder to provide a bit more airiness and rise. Doughs made with alternative flours also tend to be stickier, so if you need to work or shape a dough with your hands, I suggest keeping a bowl of water nearby to keep your hands damp and therefore less sticky. Keto doughs also tend to stick more to baking pans, so grease those pans generously! Whenever necessary, I'll also recommend the use of parchment paper in my recipes.

It is possible to create delicious keto desserts, even if they are not 100 percent the same as their high-carb versions. It is a minor trade-off to have your dessert and keto, too!

NUT-FREE AND DAIRY-FREE KETO DESSERTS

It can be tough for those who have a nut or dairy allergy (or both) to figure out keto baking and keto desserts, because the go-to alternative flour tends to be almond and because keto desserts use copious amounts of butter and cream for those satiating, creamy textures. But don't worry, you do have options! Use sunflower seed or sesame seed flour instead of most nut flours (substituted at a 1:1 ratio).

Coconut flour is also an option if you have been cleared by your doctor to use it. Because coconut flour is a much thirstier flour, it is not a 1:1 swap for nut flours. See page 14 for general guidelines on how to swap coconut flour for other flours.

Keep in mind it is vital to source nut-free flour substitutes only from a facility that does not also process nuts to prevent cross-contamination. I find coconut oil to be the best replacement for butter (dairy), and coconut or almond milk best for cow's milk. Give the Nut-Free Pumpkin Bread (page 108) and Coconut Lime Panna Cotta (page 49) recipes a try. They are nut-free, dairy-free, and delicious.

Techniques for Keto Dessert Success

I lean toward simple keto dessert recipes. I believe you can get consistent results without complicated steps or hard-to-source ingredients, with easy tips and techniques to ensure your success.

Measure Accurately

When measuring ingredients, a digital scale provides the highest accuracy; after all, baking is a science. But many people don't have a digital scale, and I've found I can still get wonderful results using standard measuring cups and spoons. Therefore, I don't require the use of a scale.

When measuring, especially nonwheat flours, do not pack the flour too tightly. For better and consistent results, spoon the ingredients into the measuring cup instead of using the cup to scoop them.

When adding liquids to a recipe, use liquid measuring cups. The key is to put the cup on a flat surface and pour the liquid to just under the appropriate line.

Sifting Makes a Difference

Sifting may seem unnecessary, especially when alternative flours are labeled "finely milled." However, it can make a remarkable difference in the outcome of your baking.

Sifting removes the coarse pieces in nut flours, which can negatively affect the texture of the final product. It's a necessary step when working with dense flours such as almond and hazelnut because they tend to have clumps and large nut pieces. Unless the recipe states otherwise, measure and then sift for the best results.

Temper Liquids Well

Tempering is required to combine ingredients at different temperatures. The goal of tempering is to slowly introduce the hot ingredient into the cold ingredient, so that the temperature of the mixture gradually rises and becomes more compatible with the temperature of the hot ingredient. If you combine two ingredients of vastly different temperatures too quickly, the mixture can curdle, seize, split, or get lumps.

Whip It Good

Learning how to whip your ingredients properly will prove to be a worthwhile investment, especially when it comes to egg whites and cream.

Heavy cream must be cold when whipped. Chilling both the bowl and whisk beforehand will speed the process.

To achieve the fullest volume when whipping egg whites, use fresh eggs and separate the yolks from the whites when cold. Then allow the whites to come to room temperature. If you get any yolk in the whites, they will not whip, so be sure to separate your eggs carefully.

Cool and Store Desserts Properly

Allowing your keto baked goods to cool before cutting into them is crucial because they can be on the crumblier side. In other words, while they're piping hot from the oven, they may lose some of their structural integrity if you try dividing them. Storing foods properly is key in any type of cooking, but because these recipes generally use a higher amount of fat and dairy and therefore have a shorter shelf life than their high-carb counterparts, proper storage is even more crucial. I have provided storage instructions with each recipe.

How to Use This Book

My goal when developing recipes for this book was to make the recipes easy and as similar to their high-carb counterparts as possible.

Not every recipe will meet the strict and ideal macros ratio of 70 percent fat, 25 percent protein, 5 percent carbs. However, you can still enjoy these keto desserts by balancing the rest of your meals for the day through careful planning. Know, though, that these recipes will always be much lower in net carbs than non-keto desserts.

Carb Counts

Net carbs are the carbs absorbed by the body. To calculate net carbs in whole foods, subtract the fiber content from the total number of carbohydrates. All the recipes in this book note net carbs in grams per serving. The recipes also note carb macro percentages, which are calculated from the number of net carbs.

Sweetener Levels

Because this cookbook relies more on whole foods and less on artificial sweeteners, I have provided, whenever possible, two amounts of sweetener—standard and less sweet. My advice is to aim for the "less sweet" amount, but you can switch to the standard amount if you find the recipe's not sweet enough. Keep in mind that when first embarking on a keto diet, your taste buds will prefer more sweetener, but as you progress, you will find you need less. Listen to your body in choosing the level of sweetness that works best for you.

Recipe Tips

Most recipes include tips that provide a little extra information and assistance. These tips include:

INGREDIENT TIP. This tip assists you in selecting ingredients and understanding how to work with them.

KEEP IN MIND. This tip offers advice to ensure the success of your final product.

SPICE IT UP. This tip offers suggestions for garnishes or decorations.

VARIATION TIP. This tip presents ingredient swaps to create a different flavor profile or presentation or to make a recipe allergen free.

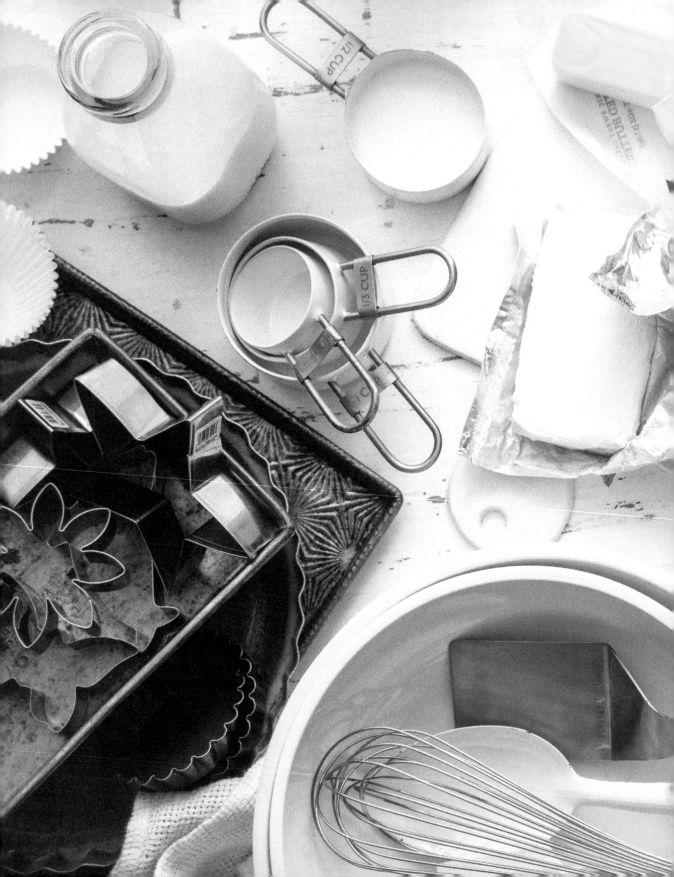

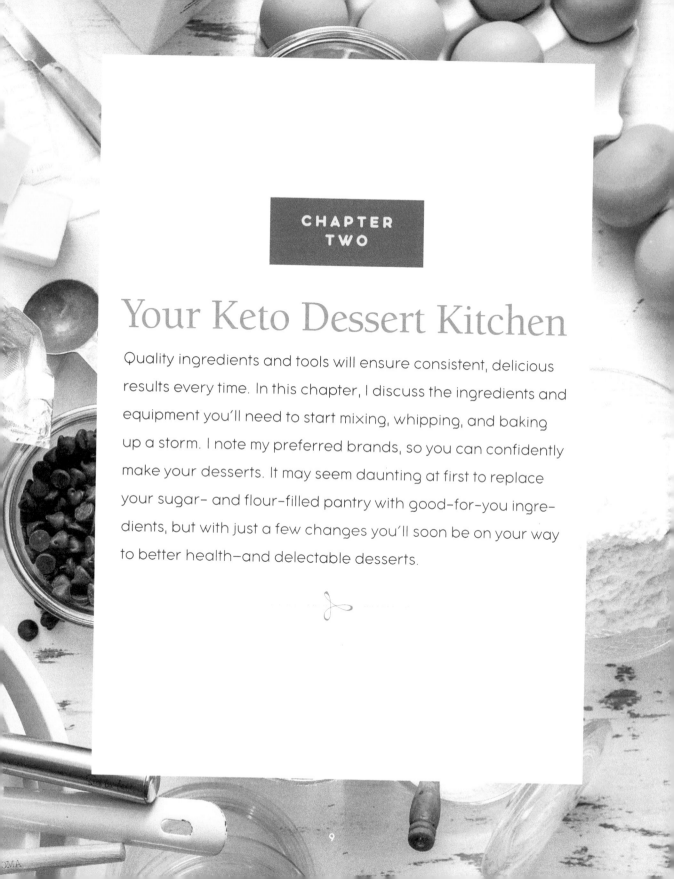

Your Keto Dessert Kitchen

Quality ingredients and tools will ensure consistent, delicious results every time. In this chapter, I discuss the ingredients and equipment you'll need to start mixing, whipping, and baking up a storm. I note my preferred brands, so you can confidently make your desserts. It may seem daunting at first to replace your sugar- and flour-filled pantry with good-for-you ingredients, but with just a few changes you'll soon be on your way to better health—and delectable desserts.

Eggs

Eggs play an important role in keto desserts as a binder, thickener, and rising agent. I recommend USDA grade AA or A large, pasture-raised eggs. For best results, use fresh eggs, and bring them to room temperature to help desserts rise and emulsify. A shortcut to bring cold eggs to room temperature is to let them sit in a bowl of hot water for 5 minutes.

Fats and Oils

Fats and oils play an important role in dessert-making. They provide flavor, moisture, and richness to keto desserts.

Butter

Butter adds a rich flavor and moisture to desserts. I recommend using unsalted butter in my recipes; salted butter can have an unpredictable amount of salt and more water. If possible, choose butter from grass-fed cows because it contains omega-3 fatty acids, which are great for brain function and so much more.

Coconut Oil

Coconut oil is a great option for replacing traditional oils in keto desserts. I recommend refined oil because it has a neutral taste and can withstand higher temperatures. Coconut oil is easy to work with; it's a great substitute for butter if you are wanting a dairy-free option. Just make sure to check whether the recipe calls for a solid or melted state, and substitute accordingly.

Keto-Friendly Flours and Meals

Low-carb flours have a short shelf life, so be sure to store them in airtight containers in a cool, dry place, and don't plan to keep them too long. Many people put their nut flours in the refrigerator for this very reason.

Almond Flour

Almond flour is a gluten-free flour with a mild, sweet, and nutty aroma. It is made from blanched, skinned almonds finely ground into flour. Almond flour is prized for its finely milled texture that comes closest to traditional wheat flour. It can be used alone, like in my Carrot Cake (page 94), or in combination with other alternative flours. My favorite brands are Bob's Red Mill Natural Foods ("Bob's Red Mill") and Anthony's Goods, which are found online and in most national grocery stores.

Coconut Flour

Coconut flour is made by dehydrating coconut meat and finely grinding it into a powder. It is low in carbs and high in fiber, making it a great option in keto desserts. Anthony's Goods is my favorite brand and can be sourced online.

Sunflower Seed Flour

Sunflower seed flour is a nut-free alternative flour. It is produced by grinding sunflower seeds into a powder. Despite being nut-free, it has a nutty, sweet flavor. Sunflower seed flour can be substituted one-for-one for almond flour. Store this flour in a cool, dry place. Sunflower seed flour is found online through Amazon and other retailers.

Almond Meal

Almond meal is coarser than almond flour. The meal is not a substitute for finely milled blanched almond flour. Store in a cool, dry place. Almond meal works well when making no-bake piecrusts, like my No-Bake Chocolate Raspberry Cheesecake (page 101). Trader Joe's makes excellent almond meal.

Flaxseed Meal

Grinding flaxseed produces a meal that can be used in keto baking as a flour substitute or even as an egg replacement. My preference is golden flaxseed meal, because regular flaxseed meal has a gummier texture that can make your baked goods too heavy. Golden flaxseed meal has a nutty flavor that works especially well in bread recipes, like my Bread Pudding (page 45). Flaxseed meal is in most grocery stores; golden flax is less common, but it can be sourced online or found in most natural foods stores. My favorite brands to use are Whole Foods 365 Everyday Value Organic (ground flaxseed) and Bob's Red Mill.

Pecan Meal

Pecan meal is produced when pecans are finely chopped. It adds a rich nutty flavor without the need for toasting and is delicious in recipes like my Pecan Chocolate Chip Cookies (page 65). Store pecan meal in a cool, dry place. King Arthur Flour has a delicious option you can source online.

Fruits

Certain fruits have more carbohydrates than others. Knowing which to include in keto dessert-making is critical. Eating too many net carbs can elevate your blood sugar and kick you out of ketosis.

Berries contain the lowest amount of carbs compared with other fruits. You can also enjoy the juice and zest of limes and lemons, which impart a lot of flavor. You'll need only a small amount. Dried, unsweetened coconut, and coconut cream and coconut milk, of course, can add both texture and flavor to your keto desserts as well.

Leavening Agents

Leavening agents are what make baked goods, such as cakes and breads, rise. Instead of being flat and dense, leavening agents make these foods light and airy. There are many kinds of leavening agents that work differently to create reactions while baking your sweets. In this section, I have highlighted two that will be used in the recipes in this book.

Baking Powder

Baking powder is a mixture of baking soda and cream of tartar and does not need an acid to rise. Keto recipes, just like regular recipes, require fresh baking powder for baked goods. Checking the expiration date and replacing it sooner if you live in a humid environment is key, because both baking powder and soda absorb a lot of moisture. I recommend using only gluten-free baking powder, such as Hain Pure Foods Featherweight Baking Powder.

Baking Soda

Baking soda rises when it reacts with acidic ingredients in a recipe to create carbon dioxide. This reaction is responsible for baked goods rising. It's important to only use what the recipe calls for because too much can produce a metallic, soapy flavor.

Milks, Creams, and Cheeses

In dessert-making, milks, creams, and cheeses play an important role. The recipes I am sharing use a combination of dairy and dairy-free options, giving you the flexibility to choose which one to use.

Nondairy Milks

Unsweetened almond and coconut milk are good nondairy choices on keto and can be used interchangeably in any of my recipes that call for a dairy-free milk option. The important thing to remember is to choose one with no added sugar.

Coconut Cream

Coconut cream is not the same as coconut milk. Much thicker and richer, coconut cream is what rises to the top of coconut milk. It is often used as a dairy-free alternative to heavy cream.

Heavy (Whipping) Cream

Heavy cream is a great substitute for regular milk. Unlike milk, it is very low in lactose and therefore relatively low in carbs.

Sour Cream

Like yogurt, sour cream is a fermented dairy product. It is made by fermenting heavy cream with lactic acid. In keto desserts, sour cream adds tang and richness.

Cream Cheese

Cream cheese is used in keto desserts for binding and stability. It also gives desserts a silky texture. Use the full-fat variety that comes in a block.

Mascarpone Cheese

Mascarpone is an Italian cream cheese made with heavy cream and lemon juice. The percentage of milk fat in mascarpone is higher than in cream cheese, making mascarpone richer and creamier.

SWAP IT!

Substitutions are necessary when you don't have a particular ingredient on hand, your diet doesn't permit the item specified in the recipe, or you don't like that ingredient. Not all ingredients are equally interchangeable. Some recipes offer substitutions, but here are some broad guidelines.

FATS. When interchanging fats, it is essential that you only substitute liquid for liquid or solid for solid. Melted butter can be swapped for melted coconut oil, for example, but don't substitute solid butter for melted coconut oil.

ALTERNATIVE FLOURS. Most nut or seed flours can be substituted at a 1:1 ratio for another nut or seed flour, but it's good to take into account the graininess and texture of the flour. For example, sunflower seed flour is an excellent substitute for blanched almond flour, because they are both similarly delicate in texture. Hazelnut flour and pecan meal are good substitutes for almond meal, because they share a coarser, nuttier profile.

COCONUT FLOUR. This flour can never be equally substituted for any nut flour because it is a much thirstier flour and does not have the same moisture content as nut flours. Recipes that call for the use of coconut flour have taken into consideration the need for additional moisture. When you substitute coconut flour for another flour, use only a quarter of the flour called for in the recipe and add another egg to provide moisture and structure.

SWEETENERS. Use the sweetener of your choice in the amount listed in all of the recipes in this book, with the exception of erythritol-stevia blends. Stevia is much sweeter, so you should use half of what is listed in the recipe.

Natural Flavoring Agents

The use of natural flavoring agents in keto desserts provides a burst of flavor that helps enhance these recipes. Natural flavors are food flavorings derived from plants or animals and nothing else. Avoid any flavor enhancers that add fillers.

Unsweetened Chocolate and Cocoa Powder

Unsweetened baking chocolate and cocoa powder are naturally sugar-free, and both add rich chocolate flavor without adding sugar. Baking chocolate can be added to recipes by melting or folding in shaved pieces to the batter. Natural unsweetened cocoa powder has an intense, bitter chocolate flavor. Baker's and Ghirardelli have great unsweetened baking chocolate, and Ghirardelli, Whole Foods 365 Everyday Value, and Hershey's make excellent unsweetened cocoa powder.

Extracts

All-natural extracts can intensify or add flavor without affecting your macros much. Look for brands that make both natural and water-soluble versions. Nature's Flavors uses only organic flavorings and has a category of keto-friendly extracts low in carbs. Some of my favorites include:

* Lemon extract, which can help boost the lemony flavor in recipes, especially when used with freshly grated lemon zest.

* Orange extract, which introduces a bright flavor to recipes. It works well in citrus-based recipes, of course, or when you want to add a nice, sharp twist to your desserts. I love adding a little orange extract to my pumpkin pies—it's unexpected, and delicious!

* Vanilla extract, which is a favorite in all dessert-making. Vanilla enhances all the flavors in sweet recipes, and if it is left out, the final product can taste flat and bland.

Spices

Spices play an essential role in dessert-making. The use of high-quality spices can make the difference between an okay dessert and an amazing one. Source fresh spices from a reputable brand. I recommend you store your spices in a cool, dry place and replace them often. Some of my favorites include:

* Cinnamon, obviously! This aromatic spice adds a warm depth.

* Ground ginger. The powdered ground version is so much easier than chopping the fresh root. With a sweet and spicy flavor profile, ginger is excellent for all fall- and winter-inspired cakes, cookies, and quick breads.

* Nutmeg. The spicy, sweet taste gives desserts such as Pumpkin Pie (page 124) a fullness of flavor.

Salt

Although adding salt to desserts may seem counterintuitive, salt actually enhances the sweetness in a dish and even helps block bitterness. Salt adds fullness to a recipe and, when missing, makes the recipe taste flat. I prefer using a fine sea salt rather than regular table salt, which is heavily processed and void of many minerals. I also like sprinkling coarse sea salt flakes, like Maldon, on certain desserts to finish them.

Sweeteners

In these recipes, you'll notice I favor erythritol blends as my sweetener of choice. This sugar alcohol, found naturally in most fruits and vegetables, does not get metabolized by the body and therefore has no effect on blood sugar levels. Erythritol gets absorbed in the small intestine, bypassing the colon, and so is not counted in the net carbs of the recipes.

I primarily use Lakanto Monkfruit Sweetener, an erythritol–monk fruit blend. Monk fruit gets its sweetness from antioxidants called mogrosides, instead of fructose or sucrose. It is a wonderful, all-natural sugar substitute with zero calories and zero glycemic index impact. I also enjoy using Swerve, an erythritol-oligosaccharides blend.

Allulose

Allulose is another sweetener I use in a few recipes in this book. It is a rare sugar found naturally in a small number of fruits. Unlike most sugar substitutes, allulose is not a sugar alcohol. Because the body doesn't metabolize allulose, it does not raise blood sugar or insulin levels and provides minimal calories. I like using allulose when making caramel sauce because it does not crystallize when it cools. It is, however, 30 percent less sweet than table sugar, so you need to use a bit more in recipes to get the same level of sweet- ness. I recommend the Anthony's Goods brand of allulose, which can be found online.

Confectioners' Sweeteners

Used primarily in making frosting and icings, powdered sweeteners or confectioners' sugar substitute is finely ground sweetener. Because of its fine texture, a powdered sweetener is twice as sweet as granulated. Both Lakanto and Swerve have excellent powdered formulations. Make your own confectioners' sweetener by grinding up granulated sweetener in a blender or coffee grinder and then passing it through a fine sieve.

Granulated Sweeteners

When it comes to choosing granulated sweeteners, you have a few options. Lakanto and Swerve are the gold standard in my mind. Both these brands have brown sugar formulations as well. If you prefer an erythritol-stevia combination, then Pyure is what I recommend. However, if using a stevia blend, you will need to use half the amount called for in the recipe because it is twice as sweet.

SWEETENERS TO AVOID

I believe it's best to avoid the following sweeteners in keto baking and dessert-making.

ASPARTAME (such as Equal and NutraSweet) and **saccharine** (such as Sweet'N Low) should be avoided because they are not natural substitutes and have been reported to cause health problems.

MALTODEXTRIN sounds like another zero-calorie sugar substitute, but it is actually a highly processed sweetener produced from starchy plants. This one contains the same number of calories and carbs as regular sugar. No thanks!

SUCRALOSE, the ingredient found in brands like Splenda, can produce harmful compounds when exposed to high temperatures and in some individuals cause an insulin spike despite having zero carbs and calories.

XYLITOL, a sugar alcohol, is as sweet as regular sugar and does not raise blood sugar levels. However, it can cause digestive problems. It's also extremely toxic for pets, so I don't keep it in my house. Ever.

Thickeners and Binders

Thickeners and binders are needed in dessert-making to help with structure and texture. Because not all are keto-friendly, here are those I recommend:

Gelatin

Gelatin can be used as a thickener in custards, gummy candies, panna cotta, and puddings. Gelatin comes in two forms—powdered and sheet. Both work well. Four sheets of leaf gelatin equals 1 tablespoon of powdered gelatin.

Psyllium Husk Powder

The husk of the seed of the psyllium plant contains a soluble fiber that, when mixed with liquids, produces a thick gel. This gel provides structure and volume in the absence of gluten. Try the NOW foods brand found in natural foods stores and online.

Xanthan Gum

Xanthan gum is a binder that works well to stabilize keto desserts in the absence of gluten. It makes the dough sticky and traps the bubbles created by the leavening agents, helping it to rise better. Adding a little xanthan gum will make your baked goods less crumbly and will give cookies and brownies a slight chewy texture. You will only need a very small amount, ½ teaspoon or less, because a little goes a long way. You may be able to find xanthan gum in large grocery stores in the gluten-free section or through online retailers.

Your Kitchen

Having the proper tools for keto dessert-making is key. Thankfully, you probably already own most of what I am recommending.

The Essentials

SQUARE BAKING PAN. An 8-by-8-inch square pan is the perfect size for making lots of keto desserts like bars and brownies. You'll get 16 portions out of this size baking pan.

BAKING SHEET. Investing in a few good baking sheets will make dessert-making easier. I like using one that is 12-by-17-inches, but your oven's capacity will help determine the size that will work best for you. Cookie sheets are not rimmed all around, whereas baking sheets are. I favor baking sheets because they work well for cookies as well as other baked goods.

HIGH-POWERED BLENDER. Having a high-powered blender will make smoothies a delicious breeze. It will also make popsicles and many other desserts faster and easier to prepare. I recommend the Vitamix Explorian blender for its many functions and high speed.

CAKE PAN. A set of 8-inch round nonstick cake pans are ideal for making multilayer cakes. I recommend the Calphalon brand for its heavy-gauge steel core, making it a great heat conductor and durable. The nonstick finish releases cakes easily and intact.

COFFEE GRINDER. Although you can purchase psyllium husk powder, I find it is still not ground finely enough. I recommend, then, that you grind it further in a coffee grinder. A spice grinder or a mortar and pestle work, too, but you will get faster results with a coffee grinder.

ELECTRIC HAND MIXER. Having an electric hand mixer will make blending much easier and produce consistent results. They are economical and portable, and they produce results similar to those of a stand mixer.

LOAF PAN. A 9-by-5-inch loaf pan is vital for making keto quick breads or pound cakes. I am partial to metal loaf pans because they conduct heat better. Glass pans, I find, can cause the loaves to be soggy. I really like the Nordic Ware 1.5-pound loaf pan because it has a great nonstick surface.

MEASURING CUPS AND SPOONS. Measuring tools are vital in dessert-making. Having clear liquid measuring cups, like the classic Pyrex glass ones, with graduated markers is necessary for accuracy. For dry ingredients, a measuring cup set is key.

MIXING BOWLS. Mixing bowls come in different sizes and materials. The recipe will determine which to use. Some factors to consider when choosing the bowl to use will include capacity and whether it can be safely put in the microwave, dishwasher, or freezer.

SILICONE MOLDS. There are a few different sizes of molds called for in this book, including silicone 1-ounce and 4-ounce molds. Ice cube trays and ramekins can be used in their place, but having a couple of different types of molds on hand will make dessert-making all the more fun.

NONSTICK MUFFIN PAN. A 12-cup nonstick muffin pan affords automatic portion control. What's great with a nonstick variety is you don't always have to use paper liners if you butter or grease the cups properly.

PIE DISH. Pie dishes can be made of glass, ceramic, or metal. Personally, I like the presentation a ceramic pie dish brings to the table. I recommend a 9-inch dish for baking or serving.

HEAVY-BOTTOMED SAUCEPAN. It's best to use a heavy-bottomed saucepan for the sauce and custard recipes. The thicker base tends to distribute heat more evenly than a thin saucepan, which is more prone to hot spots that will more easily end in burned food. I recommend Cuisinart Chef's Classic Stainless Saucepan in the 1½-quart size. It's one to turn to often in keto dessert-making.

SIFTER. I recommend using a sifter in the majority of my nut-flour recipes to help break up any clumps and to remove any large pieces of nuts and skin left behind. I recommend choosing a stainless steel 3-cup capacity sifter.

Upgrades and Nice-to-Haves

COOKIE SCOOPS. Cookie scoops may not be essential, but they can help ensure uniform sizes and portions. A small cookie scoop holds a little less than 1 ounce of dough and produces a baked cookie about 2 inches in diameter. A medium scoop holds about 1.25 ounces of dough and makes a 3-inch cookie, whereas a large scoop holds 2.25 ounces of dough and produces a 4-inch cookie. In the recipes with 1 tablespoon-size cookies, a small 1-ounce scoop works well.

PASTRY BAG AND PIPING TIPS. A pastry bag with assorted tips makes decorating your creations fun and easy! A pastry bag can also help create perfectly portioned treats and be used to drizzle cookies and bars with just the right amount of icing.

STAND MIXER. Stand mixers will make nut flour–based batters smooth quickly. They also do a fantastic job in creaming butter and cream cheese without much effort. My favorite is one of the KitchenAid Artisan Stand Mixers.

Troubleshooting Your Keto Desserts

Q. Why did my keto dessert have a cooling aftertaste?

A cooling aftertaste is not uncommon in recipes with erythritol, a natural sugar alcohol. Consider using a monk fruit–erythritol blend and reducing the amount of sweetener when the option is given in a recipe.

Q. My keto cakes and cookies are grainy and dense. How do I fix the texture?

Nut flour can be heavier than traditional wheat flours. Always measure carefully, adding tablespoonfuls to the measuring cup and then sifting.

Q. My browned butter tastes bitter, what happened?

Browning butter requires your constant attention because it can burn rather quickly, producing a bitter aftertaste instead of the fragrant nutty flavor you want. To ensure your butter does not brown too quickly, use a heavy-bottomed pan and keep a watchful eye on the butter. Take it off the fire the moment brown flakes start to form because it will continue browning once off the heat.

Q. My keto mousses didn't set properly. Why?

I would ask if you are certain you did not skip adding the gelatin or that you added the correct amount. Unflavored gelatin is vital in setting your mousse. You also need to chill the mousse completely for the time indicated, otherwise it will not fully set.

Q. Why didn't my keto cake rise?

In the majority of cases, the cake's failure to rise is a leavening issue. Make sure your baking powder has not expired. If you store your baking powder in a hot, high-humidity area, it may have expired before its expiration date. Also, check that you didn't use baking soda instead of baking powder, a common mistake. If a recipe calls for baking powder, don't use baking soda, which needs to be activated by an acid. Otherwise, the cake will certainly not rise.

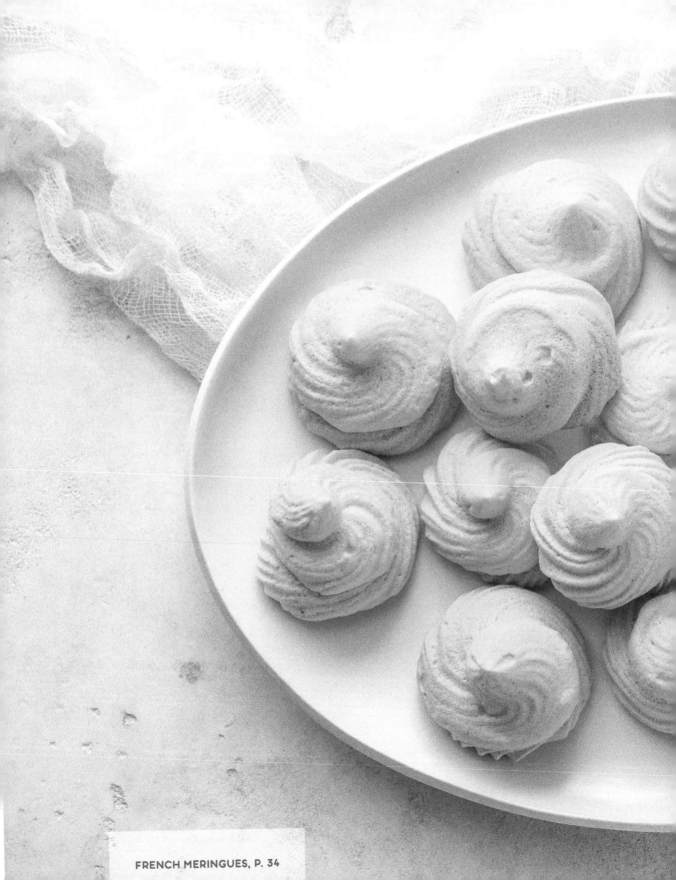

FRENCH MERINGUES, P. 34

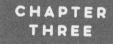

CHAPTER THREE

Candies, Confections, and Fat Bombs

Salted Caramels 24

Almond Chocolate Bark 25

Dairy-Free Chocolate Truffles 26

Pralines 27

Candied Bacon Fudge 29

Chocolate Peppermint Fudge 31

Cinnamon-Dusted Almonds 32

Chocolate-Covered Strawberries 33

French Meringues 34

Cheesecake Fat Bombs 35

Chocolate Peanut Butter
Fat Bombs 36

Cookie Dough Fat Bombs 37

Salted Caramels

PREP TIME: 3 to 5 minutes **COOK TIME:** 10 to 15 minutes **CHILL TIME:** 2 hours
EQUIPMENT: 8-by-8-inch baking pan, small saucepan, wax paper

When my keto journey began, there were many things I thought I would have to say goodbye to forever. Delicious and decadent caramels were at the top of my "impossible to make keto" list. I'm so glad I was wrong! These salted caramels are actually easy to make.

2 tablespoons unsalted butter, at room temperature

1 cup allulose

¼ teaspoon sea salt

¼ cup heavy (whipping) cream

½ teaspoon vanilla extract

1. Line the baking pan with wax paper and set aside.

2. In a small saucepan, brown the butter over medium heat for about 3 minutes, making sure to stir often while the butter browns. Add the allulose and stir until well combined. Simmer for about 7 minutes, until melted, then stir in the salt. Once it starts to bubble, add the heavy cream and vanilla and stir constantly, making sure it doesn't boil over. Once combined, reduce the heat and allow to gently simmer for about 3 minutes, until reduced slightly.

3. Remove the caramel sauce from the heat and pour it evenly into the prepared baking pan. Put into the refrigerator for a couple of hours or overnight, until cool and hardened.

4. Cut the caramel into 24 pieces and serve.

5. To store, wrap each candy in wax paper, twisting the sides closed. Put the candies in an airtight container in the refrigerator for up to 5 days. With refrigeration, the candies will become very firm but will soften at room temperature.

KEEP IN MIND: Keep a close eye on the pan once you've added the heavy cream to ensure you don't burn the sauce. The caramel will still be slightly runny until it completely cools; this is normal.

Per serving (1 piece): **Calories:** 6; **Total Fat:** 0.75g; **Total Carbohydrates:** 0g; **Net Carbs:** 0g; **Fiber:** 0g; **Protein:** 0g; **Sweetener:** 8g
Macros: Fat: 97%; **Protein:** 1%; **Carbs:** 2%

Almond Chocolate Bark

PREP TIME: 5 to 10 minutes **CHILL TIME:** 20 minutes
EQUIPMENT: medium mixing bowl, small microwave-safe bowl,
8-by-8-inch baking pan, parchment paper

Chocolate and almonds belong together. When I was growing up, my father always bought several kinds of Spanish turrón for Christmas, but my favorite was the chocolate with almonds. This almond bark is the perfect nod to that childhood after-dinner treat. It features a chocolate base, slivered almonds, and almond extract.

¾ cup coconut oil

¼ cup confectioners' erythritol–monk
  fruit blend; *less sweet: 3 tablespoons*

3 tablespoons dark cocoa powder

½ cup slivered almonds

¾ teaspoon almond extract

1. Line the baking pan with parchment paper and set aside.

2. In the microwave-safe bowl, melt the coconut oil in the microwave in 10-second intervals.

3. In the medium bowl, whisk together the melted coconut oil, confectioners' erythritol–monk fruit blend, and cocoa powder until fully combined. Stir in the slivered almonds and almond extract.

4. Pour the mixture into the prepared baking pan and spread evenly. Put the pan in the freezer for about 20 minutes, or until the chocolate bark is solid.

5. Once the chocolate bark is solid, break apart into 15 roughly even pieces to serve.

6. Store the chocolate bark in an airtight container in the freezer. Allow to slightly thaw about 5 minutes before eating. Thaw only what you will be eating.

VARIATION TIP: Get creative with this recipe! Change up the extract and nuts for different flavors.

Per serving (1 piece): Calories: 117; Total Fat: 13g; Total Carbohydrates: 1g; Net Carbs: 0g; Fiber: 1g; Protein: 1g; Sweetener: 3g
Macros: Fat: 94%; Protein: 3%; Carbs: 3%

Dairy-Free Chocolate Truffles

PREP TIME: 10 minutes **COOK TIME:** 5 minutes **CHILL TIME:** 40 minutes
EQUIPMENT: medium airtight container for chilling, small saucepan, 12-by-17-inch baking sheet, small cookie scoop (optional), parchment paper

These dairy-free chocolate truffles are beyond rich. If you prefer, you could make them with a high-quality butter instead of coconut oil. European butter brands such as Kerrygold and Plugra are great and easy to find.

¼ cup full-fat coconut milk

5 ounces sugar-free dark chocolate, finely chopped

1 tablespoon solid coconut oil, at room temperature

¼ cup unsweetened cocoa powder, for coating

1. Line the baking sheet with parchment paper and set aside.

2. In the small saucepan, heat the coconut milk over medium heat for about 3 minutes, until hot. Stir in the chocolate and let sit in the coconut milk until beginning to melt. When most of the chocolate has softened, stir carefully with a whisk until all of the chocolate is melted and the texture is smooth and glossy. Add the coconut oil and stir gently until combined.

3. Transfer the mixture to the medium airtight container and refrigerate until firm and set, about 30 minutes.

4. Using a small cookie scoop or spoon, scoop out the truffles, about 1 inch in diameter each, and shape lightly in your hands. Move quickly, and only lightly touch the chocolate or it will begin to melt in your hands.

5. Roll the truffles in the cocoa powder and place on the lined baking sheet. Refrigerate for another 10 minutes to set before serving.

6. Store leftovers in an airtight container in the refrigerator for up to 3 days or freeze for up to 3 weeks.

KEEP IN MIND: When mixing the melted chocolate in the coconut milk, be careful not to stir too vigorously. If you overmix, the chocolate may seize, becoming grainy and rough.

Per serving (1 truffle): **Calories:** 74; **Total Fat:** 6g; **Total Carbohydrates:** 3g; **Net Carbs:** 1g; **Fiber:** 2g; **Protein:** 2g; **Sweetener:** 0g
Macros: Fat: 77%; **Protein:** 8%; **Carbs:** 15%

Pralines

PREP TIME: 5 minutes **COOK TIME:** 15 minutes, plus 20 minutes to cool
EQUIPMENT: silicone spatula, 9-inch skillet, 12-by-17-inch baking sheet, parchment paper

New Orleans is one of my favorite annual trips, not least because of the city's well-deserved reputation for pralines. This keto-friendly version means I can visit the Big Easy without fear of temptation.

4 tablespoons (½ stick) unsalted butter, at room temperature

¼ cup granulated erythritol–monk fruit blend

1½ cups pecan halves

½ teaspoon salt

2 tablespoons heavy (whipping) cream

1. Line the baking sheet with parchment paper and set aside.

2. In the skillet, melt the butter over medium-high heat. Using the silicone spatula, stir in the erythritol–monk fruit blend and combine well, making sure to dissolve the sugar in the butter. Stir in the pecan halves and salt.

3. Once the pecans are completely covered in the glaze, add the heavy cream and quickly stir. When the heavy cream bubbles and evaporates, remove from the heat immediately. Quickly spoon the clusters of 4 to 5 pecan halves each onto the prepared baking sheet and allow to fully cool and set, 15 to 20 minutes, before enjoying.

4. Store leftovers in an airtight container on the counter or in the refrigerator for up 5 days.

KEEP IN MIND: Keep a close watch so the mixture does not burn once you add the heavy cream. Everything moves very quickly after this step.

Per serving (1 cluster): Calories: 85; Total Fat: 9g; Total Carbohydrates: 1g; Net Carbs: 0g; Fiber: 1g; Protein: 1g; Sweetener: 3g
Macros: Fat: 91%; Protein: 3%; Carbs: 6%

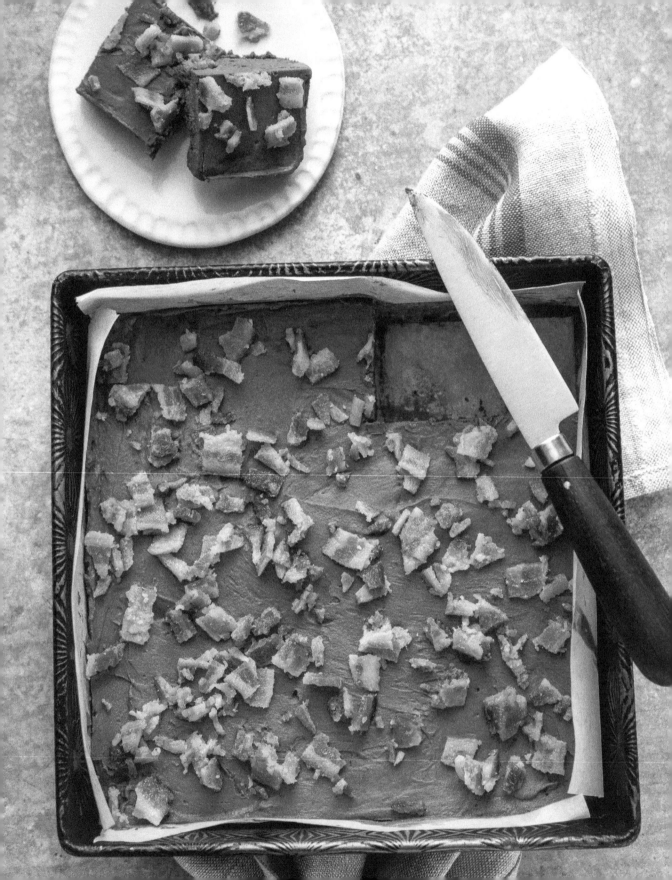

Candied Bacon Fudge

MAKES 24 BARS

PREP TIME: 10 minutes COOK TIME: 40 minutes CHILL TIME: 30 minutes
EQUIPMENT: medium shallow mixing bowl, medium mixing bowl, electric mixer, 12-by-17-inch baking sheet, 8-by-8-inch baking pan, small microwave-safe bowl, aluminum foil, parchment paper

The only thing better than bacon is candied bacon. The pairing of sweet chocolate fudge and salty bacon can't be beat. Trust me—once you try this candied bacon, you'll want to crumble it on top of everything, like my Peanut Butter Cake Bars on page 83. If you have a nut allergy, feel free to omit the pistachios—the fudge will still be delicious!

½ cup granulated erythritol–monk fruit blend

6 bacon slices

8 tablespoons (1 stick) unsalted butter, at room temperature

4 ounces unsweetened baking chocolate, coarsely chopped

1 cup confectioners' erythritol–monk fruit blend; *less sweet: ½ cup*

8 ounces full-fat cream cheese, at room temperature

¼ cup dark cocoa powder

1 teaspoon vanilla extract

1 cup chopped pistachios

1. Preheat the oven to 350°F. Line the baking sheet with aluminum foil. Line the baking pan with parchment paper and set aside.

2. In the shallow mixing bowl, put the granulated erythritol–monk fruit blend and dip the bacon slices into it to evenly coat both sides. Place the coated bacon on the prepared baking sheet and bake for 30 to 40 minutes, or until fully cooked. Once cooled, break into smaller pieces and set aside.

3. In the small microwave-safe bowl, melt the butter and baking chocolate in the microwave in 30-second intervals, then set aside.

4. In the medium mixing bowl, using an electric mixer on medium high, mix the confectioners' erythritol–monk fruit blend, cream cheese, dark cocoa powder, and vanilla until well combined, stopping and scraping the bowl once or twice, as needed. Add the melted chocolate mixture and combine until fully incorporated. Fold in three-quarters of the candied bacon and the chopped pistachios.

········▶

5. Spread the batter into the prepared baking pan. Sprinkle the remaining candied bacon on top of the fudge.

6. Put the baking pan in the freezer for about 30 minutes or until the fudge firms. Cut the fudge into 24 squares and serve.

7. Store the fudge in the refrigerator for up to 5 days or freeze for up to 3 weeks.

KEEP IN MIND: When cutting the fudge, run the knife under warm water and wipe it clean between cuts to keep the fudge from sticking to your knife.

Per serving (1 piece): Calories: 141; Total Fat: 13g; Total Carbohydrates: 4g; Net Carbs: 2g; Fiber: 2g; Protein: 3g; Sweetener: 4g
Macros: Fat: 81%; Protein: 9%; Carbs: 10%

Chocolate Peppermint Fudge

PREP TIME: 10 minutes **COOK TIME:** 5 minutes **CHILL TIME:** 30 minutes
EQUIPMENT: large mixing bowl, electric mixer, 8-by-8-inch baking pan,
small microwave-safe bowl, parchment paper

Nothing quite says Christmas like peppermint. Combine it with chocolate and you have a classic pairing. This fudge is perfectly creamy, and it's easy to make. Once December rolls around, these are a staple in my house!

8 tablespoons (1 stick) unsalted butter, at room temperature

4 ounces unsweetened baking chocolate, coarsely chopped

1 cup confectioners' erythritol–monk fruit blend; *less sweet: ½ cup*

8 ounces full-fat cream cheese, at room temperature

¼ cup dark cocoa powder

1 teaspoon vanilla extract

1½ teaspoons peppermint extract

1. Line the baking pan with parchment paper.

2. In the microwave-safe bowl, melt the butter and baking chocolate in the microwave in 30-second intervals, then set aside.

3. In the large mixing bowl, using an electric mixer on medium high, mix the confectioners' erythritol–monk fruit blend, cream cheese, cocoa powder, vanilla, and peppermint extract until well combined, stopping and scraping the bowl once or twice, as needed. Add the melted chocolate mixture and mix until fully incorporated.

4. Evenly spread the batter into the prepared baking pan. Put the baking pan in the freezer for about 30 minutes, or until the fudge firms. Cut the fudge into 24 squares and serve.

5. Store the fudge in an airtight container in the refrigerator for up to 5 days or freeze for up to 3 weeks.

VARIATION TIP: Not a fan of peppermint? Swap the peppermint extract for orange to make a chocolate orange fudge.

Per serving (1 piece): Calories: 99; **Total Fat:** 10g; **Total Carbohydrates:** 2g; **Net Carbs:** 1g; Fiber: 1g; Protein: 1g; Sweetener: 8g
Macros: **Fat:** 87%; **Protein:** 6%; **Carbs:** 7%

Cinnamon-Dusted Almonds

MAKES 2½ CUPS

PREP TIME: 5 minutes COOK TIME: 45 minutes, plus 20 minutes to cool
EQUIPMENT: 2 large mixing bowls, small mixing bowl, electric mixer, 9-by-13-inch baking sheet,
parchment paper

Almonds make a great snack because their high fat content keeps you satiated for a long time. But plain almonds can become boring. These cinnamon-dusted, mildly sweet almonds are anything but.

2½ cups whole raw almonds

2 tablespoons unsalted butter, melted

1 large egg white

½ teaspoon vanilla extract

¼ cup brown or golden erythritol–monk fruit blend; *less sweet: 2 tablespoons*

1 teaspoon ground cinnamon

¼ teaspoon sea salt

1. Preheat the oven to 275°F. Line the baking sheet with parchment paper and set aside.

2. In a large bowl, toss the almonds in the melted butter.

3. In another large bowl, using an electric mixer on medium high, lightly beat the egg white for about 1 minute, until frothy. Add the vanilla to the egg white and mix until just combined. Add the almonds and stir until well coated.

4. In the small bowl, combine the brown erythritol–monk fruit blend, cinnamon, and salt and sprinkle over the nut mixture. Toss to coat and spread evenly on the prepared baking sheet.

5. Bake for 45 minutes, stirring occasionally, until golden.

6. Allow to cool fully, 15 to 20 minutes, before eating.

7. Store in an airtight container at room temperature for up to 1 week.

VARIATION TIP: Replace the cinnamon with 1 tablespoon of cocoa powder to make chocolate-dusted almonds.

Per serving (¼ cup): Calories: 384; Total Fat: 34g; Total Carbohydrates: 13g; Net Carbs: 5g; Fiber: 8g; Protein: 13g; Sweetener: 8g
Macros: Fat: 74%; Protein: 12%; Carbs: 14%

Chocolate-Covered Strawberries

MAKES 15

PREP TIME: 10 minutes **COOK TIME:** 5 minutes **CHILL TIME:** 15 minutes
EQUIPMENT: 12-by-17-inch baking sheet, small microwave-safe bowl, parchment paper

Who can deny the irresistible combination of chocolate and strawberries? They're rich, flavorful, and oh so pretty. These strawberries would make the perfect ending to a Valentine's Day dinner . . . or any dinner, any day of the week. You can use any brand of sugar-free dark chocolate chips, but my favorite brand is Lily's.

5 ounces sugar-free dark chocolate chips
1 tablespoon vegetable
 shortening or lard

15 medium whole strawberries, fresh
 or frozen

1. Line the baking sheet with parchment paper and set aside.

2. In the microwave-safe bowl, combine the chocolate and shortening. Melt in the microwave in 30-second intervals, stirring in between.

3. Dip the strawberries into the melted chocolate mixture and place them on the prepared baking sheet.

4. Put the strawberries in the freezer for 10 to 15 minutes to set before serving.

5. Store leftovers in an airtight container in the refrigerator for up to 3 days.

INGREDIENT TIP: If you're using lard, be sure to use high-quality leaf lard, which has little to no "porky" flavor—not something you want in your chocolate-covered strawberries!

Per serving (3 strawberries): **Calories:** 217; **Total Fat:** 18g; **Total Carbohydrates:** 11g; **Net Carbs:** 6g; **Fiber:** 5g; **Protein:** 4g; **Sweetener:** 0g
Macros: Fat: 73%; **Protein:** 8%; **Carbs:** 19%

French Meringues

PREP TIME: 20 minutes **COOK TIME:** 2 hours
EQUIPMENT: large mixing bowl, rubber spatula, electric mixer, 12-by-17-inch baking sheet, parchment paper, cooling rack, pastry bag, French star tip

French meringues take patience but are easy to make. Because they don't freeze or keep well, I recommend cooking them when there's little chance of having leftovers.

4 large egg whites

¼ teaspoon cream of tartar

¼ teaspoon sea salt

½ cup granulated erythritol-monk fruit blend

¼ cup powdered erythritol-monk fruit blend

½ teaspoon vanilla extract

1. Preheat the oven to 200°F. Line the baking sheet with parchment paper and set aside.

2. In the large bowl, using an electric mixer on medium, beat the egg whites, cream of tartar, and salt for 1 to 2 minutes, until foamy and the egg whites just begin to turn opaque.

3. Continue to whip the egg whites, adding in the granulated and powdered erythritol–monk fruit blend about 1 teaspoon at a time and scraping the bowl once or twice.

4. Once all the erythritol–monk fruit blend has been added, increase the mixer speed to high and whip for 5 to 7 minutes, until the meringue is glossy and very stiff. Using a rubber spatula, gently fold in the vanilla.

5. Scoop the meringue into the pastry bag fitted with a French star tip and pipe 2-inch-diameter kisses onto the prepared baking sheet. Alternatively, spoon the meringue onto the sheet for a more organic shape.

6. Bake for 2 hours, or until crisp and lightly browned. Allow to cool completely on the cooling rack before serving. Leftovers can be stored in an airtight, nonporous container at room temperature for about 1 week.

KEEP IN MIND: To ensure stiff egg whites, rub a cut lemon around the inside of the bowl and wipe off excess moisture before whipping the whites.

Per serving (3 meringues): Calories: 8; Total Fat: 0g; Total Carbohydrates: 0g; Net Carbs: 0g; Fiber: 0g; Protein: 2g; Sweetener: 14g
Macros: Fat: 3%; Protein: 88%; Carbs: 9%

Cheesecake Fat Bombs

MAKES 30

PREP TIME: 10 minutes **CHILL TIME:** 1 hour
EQUIPMENT: large mixing bowl, electric mixer, pastry bag, 1-ounce-cavity silicone candy molds or mini cupcake liners

With just a few basic ingredients and very little effort, you can have little heavenly bites of frozen cheesecake. These bites will quickly satiate your hunger, and you can easily customize their flavor (see tip).

8 ounces full-fat cream cheese, at room temperature

8 tablespoons (1 stick) unsalted butter, at room temperature

3 tablespoons confectioners' erythritol–monk fruit blend

3 tablespoons coconut oil

½ teaspoon vanilla extract

1. In the large mixing bowl, using an electric mixer on high, beat the cream cheese and butter for 2 to 3 minutes, until light and fluffy, stopping and scraping the bowl once or twice, as needed. Add the confectioners' erythritol–monk fruit blend, coconut oil, and vanilla and mix until well combined.

2. Scoop the mixture into a pastry bag and pipe into the molds or cupcake liners. Put the molds in the freezer for 1 hour to firm. Pop out the fat bombs to serve.

3. Store in an airtight container in the freezer for up to 3 weeks.

VARIATION TIP: Have fun with the cheesecake flavors! Add ¼ cup of pureed fresh or frozen strawberries after beating the cream cheese and butter together for a strawberry cheesecake fat bomb, or mix in 2 tablespoons of lemon juice and 1 teaspoon of finely grated lemon zest for a lemony version.

Per serving (1 piece): **Calories:** 65; **Total Fat:** 7g; **Total Carbohydrates:** 0g; **Net Carbs:** 0g; **Fiber:** 0g; **Protein:** 0g; **Sweetener:** 1g
Macros: Fat: 95%; **Protein:** 3%; **Carbs:** 2%

Chocolate Peanut Butter Fat Bombs

MAKES 24

PREP TIME: 5 minutes **COOK TIME:** 5 minutes **CHILL TIME:** 30 minutes
EQUIPMENT: small microwave-safe bowl, 1-ounce-cavity silicone candy molds

These chocolate and peanut butter fat bombs are indulgent guilt killers. They'll remind you of their sugar-laden counterpart but will give you an energy boost instead of a crash. If you're not a fan of peanut butter, use your favorite nut butter.

½ cup no-sugar-added peanut butter

½ cup coconut oil

¼ cup unsweetened cocoa powder

⅓ cup confectioners' erythritol–monk fruit blend; *less sweet:*

2½ *tablespoons*

¼ teaspoon sea salt

1. In the small microwave-safe bowl, melt the peanut butter, coconut oil, and cocoa powder in the microwave in 30-second intervals, mixing in between. Once the peanut butter mixture is completely melted, stir in the confectioners' erythritol–monk fruit blend and salt.

2. Pour the mixture into the silicone molds and put in the freezer for about 30 minutes, or until they are completely set.

3. Remove the bombs from the silicone molds to serve.

4. To store, transfer to an airtight container and put in the freezer for up to 3 weeks.

SPICE IT UP: Sprinkle the fat bombs with some flaky sea salt for a little decorative flair before putting them into the freezer to set.

Per serving (1 piece): Calories: 70; Total Fat: 7g; Total Carbohydrates: 2g; Net Carbs: 2g; Fiber: 0g; Protein: 1g; Sweetener: 3g
Macros: Fat: 90%; Protein: 1%; Carbs: 9%

Cookie Dough Fat Bombs

PREP TIME: 5 minutes **CHILL TIME:** 1 hour 15 minutes
EQUIPMENT: medium mixing bowl, electric mixer, 12-by-17-inch baking sheet, small cookie scoop (optional), parchment paper

Eating cookie dough is delightful but risky (think raw eggs). These fat bombs provide the pleasure without the danger—or the sugar! I love having them stocked in the freezer for a pick-me-up! For a nutty crunch, roll the fat bombs in chopped almonds or pecans before putting them in the refrigerator to firm up.

8 ounces full-fat cream cheese, at room temperature

8 tablespoons (1 stick) unsalted butter, at room temperature

¾ cup almond flour

½ cup granulated erythritol–monk fruit blend; *less sweet:* ¼ cup

1 teaspoon vanilla extract

¼ teaspoon sea salt

¼ cup chocolate chips

1. Line the baking sheet with parchment paper and set aside.

2. In the medium bowl, using an electric mixer on high, blend the cream cheese and butter, stopping and scraping the bowl once or twice, as needed. Add the almond flour, erythritol–monk fruit blend, vanilla, and salt and mix until fully incorporated. Fold in the chocolate chips.

3. Refrigerate the mixture for 1 hour until firm (like ice cream). Using a small cookie scoop or spoon, scoop the fat bombs into 1 tablespoon-size mounds and place onto the baking sheet. Put the baking sheet back into the refrigerator for about 15 minutes to allow the fat bombs to firm before serving.

4. To store, put in an airtight container in the refrigerator for up to 10 days or in the freezer for up to 3 weeks.

Per serving (1 piece): Calories: 124; Total Fat: 12g; Total Carbohydrates: 2g; Net Carbs: 1g; Fiber: 1g;
Protein: 2g; Sweetener: 5g
Macros: Fat: 88%; Protein: 6%; Carbs: 6%

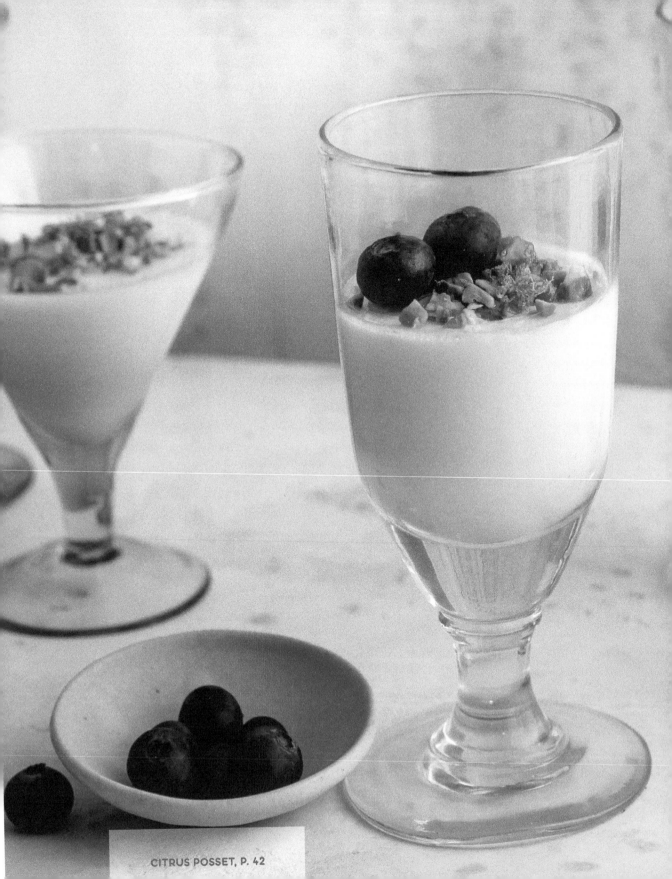

CITRUS POSSET, P. 42

CHAPTER FOUR

Custards, Puddings, and Mousses

Flan 40

Citrus Posset 42

Espresso Panna Cotta 43

Chocolate Pudding 44

Bread Pudding 45

Coconut Lime Panna Cotta 49

Mixed Berry Parfaits 50

Fresh Strawberry Mousse 52

Dairy-Free Mocha Mousse 53

Cheesecake Mousse 54

Fresh Fruit Trifle 56

Flan

PREP TIME: 5 minutes COOK TIME: 45 minutes, plus 20 minutes to cool CHILL TIME: 8 hours
EQUIPMENT: large mixing bowl, silicone spatula, small saucepan, 6 (5-ounce) ramekins,
9-by-13-inch baking pan, sieve, cooling rack

Few desserts are as synonymous with Latin culture as flan. I thought I'd never be able to pull off a keto-friendly version of this rich, eggy custard, but I am proud to say this Cuban-inspired flan has the perfect consistency and flavor. Bonus: It's a breeze to make.

2 tablespoons unsalted butter, at room temperature

1 cup allulose

3 large eggs

2 large egg yolks

½ cup granulated erythritol–monk fruit blend

2¾ cups heavy (whipping) cream

2 teaspoons vanilla extract

¼ teaspoon salt

1. Preheat the oven to 350°F. Position the rack in the center of oven.

2. In the small saucepan, brown the butter over medium heat, stirring constantly using a silicone spatula. The butter will begin to foam and bubble after 2 to 4 minutes and you should begin to see browned bits on the bottom of the pan. At this point, remove from the heat and continue to stir until the butter begins to lightly brown. Add the allulose and continue stirring over low heat for 3 to 5 minutes, until the sweetener completely dissolves and is a golden amber color.

3. Pour the sauce into the bottom of each ramekin, being sure to wiggle the dish side to side so the sauce covers the sides and bottom of the ramekins. Put the ramekins in the baking pan and set aside.

4. In the large bowl, whisk the whole eggs, egg yolks, and erythritol–monk fruit blend until combined. Gently whisk in the heavy cream, vanilla, and salt, avoiding creating a foam by whisking too vigorously.

5. Pour the custard through the sieve into the prepared ramekins. Add enough hot water to the baking pan to come halfway up the sides of the ramekins.

6. Bake for 30 minutes, or until the centers of the flans are gently set. Transfer the flans to the cooling rack to cool for 15 to 20 minutes.

7. Once cooled, cover the flans and put them in the refrigerator to chill overnight or for at least 8 hours. When ready to serve, put a plate over the top of the ramekins and flip them over to release the flans. You made need to wiggle the dish a little to ease them out. Serve and enjoy.

8. Store leftovers in an airtight container in the refrigerator for up to 3 days.

VARIATION TIP: Instead of baking small individual flans in ramekins, you could pour the whole batch of sauce followed by the batter into an 9-by-5-inch glass baking dish. Put the dish in a baking pan filled with 1 inch of hot water and bake for about 40 minutes.

Per serving: **Calories:** 468; **Total Fat:** 48g; **Total Carbohydrates:** 4g; **Net Carbs:** 4g; **Fiber:** 0g; **Protein:** 6g; **Sweetener:** 48g
Macros: Fat: 91%; **Protein:** 6%; **Carbs:** 3%

Citrus Posset

PREP TIME: 5 minutes **COOK TIME:** 10 minutes **CHILL TIME:** 6 hours
EQUIPMENT: small saucepan, 4 (¼-cup) ramekins, plastic wrap

A posset is a classic English pudding; it's luscious and custardy—but doesn't use any eggs. Instead, its velvety smooth texture is created with citrus juice. Don't adjust the amount of juice or your posset won't set properly. Instead, get creative with flavorings: Swap the orange extract for vanilla or lemon, or use only one type of citrus juice instead of both lemon and lime. Feel free to get creative with your containers too—you can use mason jars, glasses, or even pretty teacups!

2½ cups heavy (whipping) cream

½ cup granulated erythritol–monk fruit blend

¼ cup freshly squeezed lemon juice

2 tablespoons freshly squeezed lime juice

½ teaspoon orange extract

¼ teaspoon sea salt

¼ cup blueberries, for garnish (optional)

1. In the small saucepan, cook the heavy cream and erythritol–monk fruit blend over medium heat for 6 minutes, or until the sweetener has dissolved. Stir constantly so the mixture does not boil over.

2. Remove the cream mixture from the heat and stir in the lemon juice, lime juice, orange extract, and salt.

3. Pour the mixture into the ramekins and cover with plastic wrap.

4. Chill for at least 6 hours or overnight to allow the mixture to fully set before serving. Garnish with the blueberries (if using).

5. Store leftovers in an airtight container for up to 5 days in the refrigerator.

SPICE IT UP: Serve topped with lemon or lime zest (or both), whipped cream, or chopped pistachios.

Per serving: Calories: 519; Total Fat: 55g; Total Carbohydrates: 6g; Net Carbs: 6g; Fiber: 0g; Protein: 3g; Sweetener: 24g
Macros: Fat: 93%; Protein: 3%; Carbs: 4%

Espresso Panna Cotta

PREP TIME: 10 minutes **COOK TIME:** 20 minutes **CHILL TIME:** 4 hours 30 minutes
EQUIPMENT: small mixing bowl, medium saucepan, 4 (4-ounce-cavity) silicone molds, plastic wrap

Impress your guests with the perfect finale to a fancy dinner party, or spoil yourself any afternoon with this lightly coffee-flavored panna cotta. You'll find yourself making this incredibly easy and forgiving creamy dessert often.

Unsalted butter, for greasing

2 tablespoons unflavored gelatin

3 tablespoons cold water

2 cups heavy (whipping) cream

⅓ cup granulated erythritol–monk fruit blend; *less sweet: 3 tablespoons*

½ teaspoon vanilla extract

½ teaspoon espresso instant powder

⅛ teaspoon salt

1. Grease the silicone molds with butter and set aside.

2. In the small mixing bowl, dissolve the gelatin in the cold water and set aside.

3. In the medium saucepan, boil the heavy cream on medium heat. Lower the heat and simmer for about 4 minutes, until the cream begins to thicken.

4. Add the erythritol–monk fruit blend, vanilla, espresso powder, and salt. Continue to stir to combine all the ingredients. Remove from the heat and add the dissolved gelatin. Stir until the gelatin is well incorporated.

5. Pour the mixture into the molds and allow it to cool at room temperature for about 30 minutes. After cooling, cover the molds with plastic wrap and put them in the refrigerator for at least 4 hours before taking the panna cotta out of the molds. Serve cold.

6. Store leftovers in an airtight container in the refrigerator for up to 3 days.

KEEP IN MIND: To help remove the panna cotta from the molds, dip the molds in a bowl of hot water to help loosen. Greasing the silicone molds lightly and evenly will also help greatly with making the unmolding easier. Alternatively, cool the panna cotta in individual serving dishes such as ramekins to avoid the molds altogether.

Per serving: Calories: 450; Total Fat: 47g; Total Carbohydrates: 3g; Net Carbs: 3g; Fiber: 0g; Protein: 6g; Sweetener: 16g
Macros: Fat: 92%; Protein: 5%; Carbs: 3%

Chocolate Pudding

SERVES 4

PREP TIME: 5 minutes COOK TIME: 15 minutes CHILL TIME: 1 to 2 hours
EQUIPMENT: 2 medium mixing bowls, medium saucepan, sieve, plastic wrap

This rich and silky pudding is simple to make and easy to jazz up with chopped nuts or sliced berries.

2 cups heavy (whipping) cream

2 ounces unsweetened baking chocolate, coarsely chopped

1 teaspoon vanilla extract

6 large egg yolks

⅓ cup granulated erythritol–monk fruit blend

1. In the medium saucepan, heat the heavy cream over low heat for 2 to 3 minutes, until warm. Stir in the chocolate and vanilla and heat for about 3 minutes, stirring occasionally, until the chocolate has melted. Set aside to cool.

2. In a medium bowl, whisk the egg yolks and erythritol–monk fruit blend for about 2 minutes, or until the mixture is a pale yellow.

3. Once the heavy cream mixture has cooled to room temperature, 15 to 20 minutes, pour one-quarter of it into the egg mixture and whisk until well combined. Add the remaining three-quarters of the cream mixture and whisk until combined.

4. Pour the cream and egg mixture back into the saucepan. Cook over low heat, stirring constantly for 3 to 5 minutes, until the mixture begins to thicken. You'll know the pudding is thick enough when it coats the back of a spoon without dripping.

5. Pour the pudding through the sieve into another medium bowl. Put a sheet of plastic wrap directly onto the surface of the pudding to prevent a skin from forming. Completely cool the pudding in the refrigerator, about 1 to 2 hours.

6. Serve in small shallow bowls or in individual ramekins. Store leftovers in an airtight container for up to 5 days in the refrigerator.

KEEP IN MIND: If you just can't wait to eat your chocolate pudding, cool it more quickly by placing the bowl of pudding into a larger bowl filled with ice cubes.

Per serving (¼ cup): Calories: 587; Total Fat: 58g; Total Carbohydrates: 8g; Net Carbs: 6g; Fiber: 2g; Protein: 9g; Sweetener: 16g
Macros: Fat: 88%; Protein: 8%; Carbs: 6%

Bread Pudding

SERVES 12

PREP TIME: 20 minutes COOK TIME: 2 hours, plus 20 minutes to cool
EQUIPMENT: 2 large mixing bowls, medium mixing bowl, electric mixer, 2 (10-by-13-inch) baking sheets, medium saucepan, small saucepan

Bread pudding is a classic comfort dessert. This keto-friendly version is so close to the real thing it's hard to believe it has so few carbs. A decadent rum sauce further elevates it. If you plan to serve the bread pudding at the table, you can bake it in a ceramic baking dish instead of the baking sheet.

FOR THE BREAD

Unsalted butter, for greasing

6 tablespoons coconut flour

4 ounces full-fat cream cheese, at room temperature

½ cup golden flaxseed meal, re-ground in a clean coffee grinder

2 large eggs

1 tablespoon granulated erythritol–monk fruit blend

1 teaspoon baking powder

⅛ teaspoon salt

6 tablespoons heavy (whipping) cream

¼ cup water

FOR THE BREAD PUDDING

2 tablespoons unsalted butter, at room temperature, plus more for greasing

¾ cup heavy (whipping) cream

2 tablespoons water

2 large eggs

¼ cup granulated erythritol–monk fruit blend

½ teaspoon vanilla extract

⅛ teaspoon salt

FOR THE BROWN BUTTER RUM SAUCE

2 tablespoons unsalted butter, at room temperature

6 tablespoons allulose

¼ cup heavy (whipping) cream

¼ teaspoon salt

½ tablespoon dark rum or ¼ teaspoon rum extract

TO MAKE THE BREAD

1. Preheat the oven to 350°F. Grease the baking sheet with butter and set aside.

2. In a large bowl, using an electric mixer on high, mix the coconut flour, cream cheese, flaxseed meal, eggs, erythritol–monk fruit blend, baking powder, and salt until just combined, stopping and scraping the bowl once or twice, as needed. Slowly add the heavy cream and water to the batter and mix until thoroughly combined.

........⟶

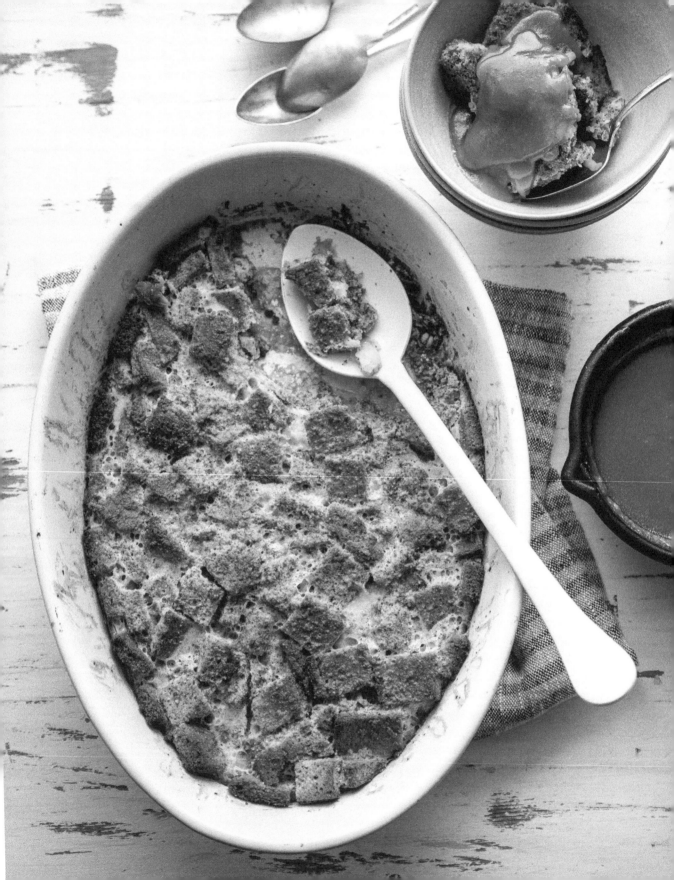

3. Pour the batter into the prepared baking sheet and bake for 30 to 35 minutes, or until lightly browned. Allow the bread to fully cool, 15 to 20 minutes, and cut into 1-inch squares. Put the cubed bread in another large mixing bowl. Leave the oven on.

TO MAKE THE BREAD PUDDING

4. Grease another baking sheet generously with butter and set aside.

5. In the medium saucepan, bring the heavy cream and water almost to a boil, then reduce the heat and add the 2 tablespoons of butter.

6. In the medium bowl, whisk the eggs, erythritol–monk fruit blend, vanilla, and salt. Temper the egg mixture by adding 3 tablespoons of the hot cream mixture to it and mixing well. Stir the remaining cream mixture into the egg mixture.

7. Pour the cream and egg mixture over the cubed bread in the large mixing bowl, toss to coat, and pour everything into the buttered baking sheet. Using a spoon, press down the bread to ensure the liquid covers it.

8. Bake for 40 to 45 minutes at 350°F or until the egg mixture has set and the top is lightly browned. Cool for 5 minutes.

9. Store leftovers in an airtight container in the refrigerator for up to 3 days.

TO MAKE THE BROWN BUTTER RUM SAUCE

10. In the small saucepan, brown the butter over medium-low heat, stirring constantly. The butter will begin to foam and bubble, and after 2 to 4 minutes, you should begin to see browned bits on the bottom of the pan. At this point, remove the pan from the heat and continue to stir until the butter begins to lightly brown to a golden amber color.

11. Add the allulose, heavy cream, and salt to the browned butter and stir until well combined. Simmer over low heat for 15 minutes. Resist the urge to stir. At the 15-minute mark, turn off the stove and add the rum. Note that the sauce will foam up when you add the rum. Stir and turn the heat to low and allow the sauce to cook for another 10 minutes without stirring. This will thicken the sauce and cook down the alcohol.

12. To serve, cut the bread pudding into 12 slices and pour the rum sauce over each slice.

13. Store leftover sauce in an airtight container in the refrigerator for up to 3 days.

KEEP IN MIND: Although the flaxseed meal comes milled, I like to run it through a clean coffee grinder for a finer texture so that the bread won't be rubbery. If you don't have a clean coffee grinder, a high-speed blender works well, too.

Per serving: **Calories:** 326; **Total Fat:** 32g; **Total Carbohydrates:** 7g; **Net Carbs:** 3g; **Fiber:** 4g; **Protein:** 5g; **Sweetener:** 11g
Macros: Fat: 85%; **Protein:** 6%; **Carbs:** 9%

Coconut Lime Panna Cotta

PREP TIME: 10 minutes **COOK TIME:** 10 minutes, plus 30 minutes to cool **CHILL TIME:** 4 hours
EQUIPMENT: small mixing bowl, medium saucepan, 4 (4-ounce-cavity) silicone molds, plastic wrap

This panna cotta is bursting with tart lime and sweet coconut flavors. Treat yourself to this simple and refreshing dessert any time you need to imagine you're on a beach. Top your panna cotta with a few fresh blueberries and some whipped cream for an extra-fancy treat!

Coconut oil, for greasing

2 tablespoons unflavored gelatin

3 tablespoons cold water

1 (13.5-ounce) can full-fat coconut milk

⅓ cup granulated erythritol–monk fruit
  blend; *less sweet: 3 tablespoons*

1 teaspoon grated lime zest

1 tablespoon freshly squeezed lime juice

½ teaspoon vanilla extract

⅛ teaspoon salt

1. Grease the molds with coconut oil and set aside.

2. In the small bowl, soften the gelatin powder in the cold water and set aside.

3. In the medium saucepan, heat the coconut milk over medium heat until boiling. Reduce the heat and simmer for a couple of minutes, until the cream begins to thicken. While stirring, add the erythritol–monk fruit blend, lime zest, lime juice, vanilla, and salt. Continue to stir to combine all the ingredients. Remove from the heat and add the dissolved gelatin. Stir until the gelatin is dissolved.

4. Pour the mixture into the prepared molds and allow them to cool at room temperature for about 30 minutes. Cover with plastic wrap and put in the refrigerator for at least 4 hours before unmolding.

5. To remove the panna cotta from the molds, dip the molds in a bowl of hot water to help loosen. Serve cold.

6. Store leftovers in an airtight container or covered with plastic wrap in the refrigerator for up to 3 days.

Per serving: Calories: 212; Total Fat: 21g; Total Carbohydrates: 3g; Net Carbs: 3g; Fiber: 0g; Protein: 5g; Sweetener: 16g
Macros: Fat: 86%; Protein: 9%; Carbs: 5%

Mixed Berry Parfaits

PREP TIME: 10 minutes COOK TIME: 10 minutes CHILL TIME: 2 hours
EQUIPMENT: 2 medium mixing bowls, small mixing bowl, medium saucepan, sieve,
4 (8-ounce) mason jars, plastic wrap

Parfait is French for "perfect." This keto version with layers of vanilla pudding and fresh fruit is exactly that! To save time, make the pudding the night before you plan to enjoy it.

FOR THE PUDDING

2 cups heavy (whipping) cream

1 teaspoon vanilla extract

6 large egg yolks

¼ cup granulated erythritol–monk fruit blend

1 tablespoon unsalted butter, at room temperature

FOR THE MIXED BERRIES

1 cup blueberries

5 strawberries, thinly sliced

1 cup raspberries

¼ cup freshly squeezed lemon juice

1 tablespoon granulated erythritol–monk fruit blend

½ cup slivered almonds, for topping

TO MAKE THE PUDDING

1. In the medium saucepan, heat the heavy cream over low heat until hot. Stir in the vanilla, then set aside to cool.

2. In a medium bowl, whisk the egg yolks, erythritol–monk fruit blend, and butter for about 2 minutes, until the mixture is a pale yellow.

3. Once the cream has cooled to the touch, pour one-quarter of the heavy cream mixture into the egg mixture and whisk until well combined. Add the remainder of the cream mixture and mix well.

4. Pour the cream and egg mixture back into the saucepan and cook over low heat, stirring continuously for about 5 minutes, or until the mixture begins to thicken. You'll know the pudding is thick enough when it coats the back of the spoon without dripping.

5. Pour the pudding through the sieve into another medium bowl. Put a sheet of plastic wrap directly onto the surface of the pudding to prevent a skin from forming. Move the pudding to the refrigerator for 1 to 2 hours to cool completely.

6. While the pudding cools, in the small bowl, combine the blueberries, strawberries, raspberries, lemon juice, and erythritol–monk fruit blend and mix.

7. Once the pudding has cooled, completely assemble the parfaits. In a mason jar or any 8-ounce glass container, add ⅓ cup of pudding and top with the berry mixture, repeating the layers until the glass is full, ending with berries. Top with slivered almonds before serving.

8. Store leftovers in an airtight container for up to 5 days in the refrigerator.

SPICE IT UP: These parfaits are perfect to set up for a brunch with a toppings bar of almonds, pistachios, sugar-free chocolate chips, whipped cream, or any of your favorite keto toppings!

Per serving (1 jar): Calories: 645; Total Fat: 61g; Total Carbohydrates: 19g; Net Carbs: 14g; Fiber: 5g; Protein: 10g; Sweetener: 15g
Macros: Fat: 83%; Protein: 6%; Carbs: 11%

Fresh Strawberry Mousse

SERVES 6

PREP TIME: 10 minutes **CHILL TIME:** 1 hour 5 minutes
EQUIPMENT: large metal mixing bowl, blender or food processor, electric mixer

When what you need is a quick dessert, this smooth strawberry mousse is perfect. The mousse features fresh strawberries, heavy cream, and a little cream cheese for stability. It's a refreshing, light, and airy treat sure to become a family favorite.

8 ounces strawberries, sliced

¼ cup granulated erythritol–monk fruit blend; *less sweet: 2 tablespoons*

½ ounce full-fat cream cheese, at room temperature

1 cup heavy (whipping) cream, divided

⅛ teaspoon vanilla extract

⅛ teaspoon salt

1. Put the large metal bowl in the freezer to chill for at least 5 minutes.

2. In a blender or food processor, puree the strawberries and erythritol–monk fruit blend. Set aside.

3. In the chilled large bowl, using an electric mixer on medium high, beat the cream cheese and ¼ cup of heavy cream until well combined, stopping and scraping the bowl once or twice, as needed. Add the vanilla and salt and mix to combine. Add the remaining ¾ cup of heavy cream and beat on high for 1 to 3 minutes, until very stiff peaks form.

4. Gently fold the puree into the whipped cream. Refrigerate for at least 1 hour and up to overnight before serving.

5. Serve in short glasses or small mason jars.

6. Store leftovers in an airtight container for up to 5 days in the refrigerator.

KEEP IN MIND: To ensure your mousse retains its structure, beat the cream mixture until very stiff before adding the strawberry puree. The mousse will deflate slightly when the puree is added, so beating it to stiff peaks will help compensate for this.

Per serving (⅙ cup): **Calories:** 157; **Total Fat:** 16g; **Total Carbohydrates:** 4g; **Net Carbs:** 3g; **Fiber:** 1g; **Protein:** 1g; **Sweetener:** 8g
Macros: Fat: 87%; **Protein:** 3%; **Carbs:** 10%

Dairy-Free Mocha Mousse

PREP TIME: 10 minutes **CHILL TIME:** 1 hour
EQUIPMENT: large metal mixing bowl, electric mixer

Coffee and chocolate lovers rejoice. This mocha mousse is easy to make and sure to please. It's perfect for any holiday. For an extra decadent touch, top the mousse with whipped cream before dusting it with cocoa powder.

1 (13.5-ounce) can coconut cream, chilled overnight

3 tablespoons granulated erythritol–monk fruit blend; *less sweet: 2 tablespoons*

2 tablespoons unsweetened cocoa powder, plus more for dusting

1 teaspoon instant espresso powder

¼ teaspoon salt

1. Put the large metal bowl in the freezer to chill for at least 1 hour.

2. In the chilled large bowl, using an electric mixer on high, combine the coconut cream (adding it by the spoonful and reserving the water that has separated), erythritol–monk fruit blend, the cocoa powder, espresso powder, and salt and beat for 3 to 5 minutes, until stiff peaks form, stopping and scraping the bowl once or twice, as needed. If the consistency is too thick, add the reserved water from the coconut cream 1 tablespoon at a time to thin.

3. Serve immediately in a cold glass, dusted with cocoa powder.

4. Store leftovers in an airtight container for up to 5 days in the refrigerator.

INGREDIENT TIP: If you can't find coconut cream, buy a few cans of full-fat coconut milk, chill it in the refrigerator overnight, then remove the cream on top and proceed with the recipe. You'll probably need five cans to get enough cream for this recipe.

Per serving (¼ cup): **Calories:** 125; **Total Fat:** 12g; **Total Carbohydrates:** 3g; **Net Carbs:** 2g; **Fiber:** 1g; **Protein:** 0g; **Sweetener:** 12g
Macros: Fat: 86%; **Protein:** 4%; **Carbs:** 10%

Cheesecake Mousse

PREP TIME: 15 minutes **CHILL TIME:** 1 hour 5 minutes
EQUIPMENT: large metal mixing bowl, small mixing bowl, electric mixer

The crumble on this no-bake dessert is so yummy, but chopped nuts and berries work as well.

FOR THE MOUSSE

2 ounces full-fat cream cheese, at room temperature

1½ cups heavy (whipping) cream, divided

¼ cup granulated erythritol–monk fruit blend; *less sweet: 2 tablespoons*

½ teaspoon vanilla extract

½ teaspoon salt

FOR THE CRUMBLE

½ cup finely milled almond flour

¼ cup coconut flour

¼ cup granulated erythritol–monk fruit blend

½ teaspoon ground cinnamon

⅛ teaspoon sea salt

4 tablespoons (½ stick) cold unsalted butter, thinly sliced

TO MAKE THE MOUSSE

1. Put the large metal bowl in the freezer to chill for at least 5 minutes.

2. In the large chilled bowl, using an electric mixer on medium high, mix the cream cheese and ¼ cup of heavy cream until well combined. Add the erythritol–monk fruit blend, vanilla, and salt and mix until just combined. Add the remaining 1¼ cups of heavy cream and beat on high for about 3 minutes, until stiff peaks form, stopping and scraping the bowl once or twice, as needed. Refrigerate for at least 1 hour and up to overnight before serving.

TO MAKE THE CRUMBLE

3. In the small bowl, combine the almond flour, coconut flour, erythritol–monk fruit blend, cinnamon, and salt. Add the sliced butter and combine using a fork until the mixture resembles coarse crumbs. Set aside until ready to serve.

4. Serve the mousse in short glasses or small mason jars topped with the crumble. Store leftovers in an airtight container for up to 5 days in the refrigerator.

Per serving (⅓ cup): Calories: 273; Total Fat: 29g; Total Carbohydrates: 3g; Net Carbs: 2g; Fiber: 1g; Protein: 3g; Sweetener: 12g
Macros: Fat: 91%; Protein: 4%; Carbs: 5%

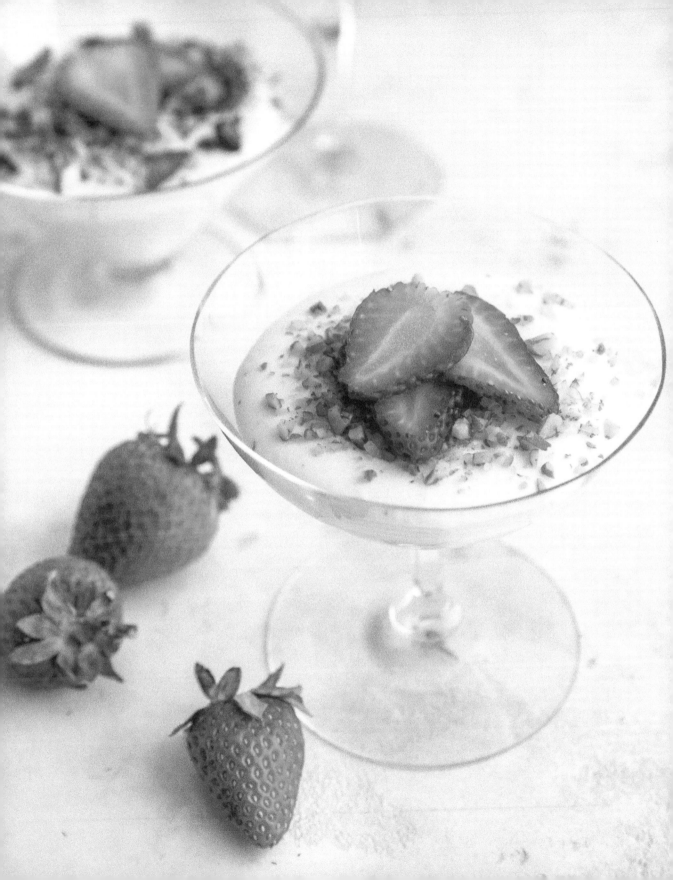

Fresh Fruit Trifle

SERVES 10

PREP TIME: 10 minutes **COOK TIME:** 40 minutes
EQUIPMENT: 2 medium mixing bowls, 3 large mixing bowls, electric mixer, 9-by-5-inch loaf pan,
9-inch trifle dish or glass bowl, parchment paper, toothpicks

This tasty trifle is a convenient option for hectic holidays because the layers can be made ahead of time, but be sure to assemble them at least an hour before serving. Save a few whole berries for the topping.

FOR THE CAKE

4 tablespoons unsalted butter, at room temperature, plus more for greasing

1¼ cups finely milled almond flour, sifted

1 teaspoon baking powder

¼ teaspoon salt

¾ cup granulated erythritol–monk fruit blend; *less sweet: ½ cup*

4 ounces full-fat cream cheese, at room temperature

1 teaspoon vanilla extract

4 large eggs, at room temperature

FOR THE FRUIT

1 cup fresh or frozen blueberries

8 ounces fresh or frozen strawberries, thinly sliced

2 tablespoons granulated erythritol–monk fruit blend;
less sweet: 1 tablespoon

½ tablespoon freshly squeezed lemon juice

FOR THE CHEESECAKE WHIPPED CREAM

2 cups heavy (whipping) cream

8 ounces full-fat cream cheese, at room temperature

¼ cup granulated erythritol–monk fruit blend; *less sweet: 2 tablespoons*

1 teaspoon vanilla extract

TO MAKE THE CAKE

1. Preheat the oven to 350°F. Grease the loaf pan with butter, line with parchment paper, and set aside.

2. In a medium bowl, combine the almond flour, baking powder, and salt. Set aside.

3. In a large bowl, using an electric mixer on high, cream the butter with the erythritol–monk fruit blend for 2 to 3 minutes, stopping and scraping the bowl once or twice, as needed, until the mixture is light and fluffy and well incorporated.

4. Add the cream cheese and vanilla and mix well. Add the eggs, one at a time, making sure to mix well after each addition. Add the dry ingredients to the wet ingredients and mix well until the batter is fully combined. Scrape the batter into the prepared loaf pan.

5. Bake for 30 to 40 minutes, until golden brown on top and a toothpick inserted into the center comes out clean. Remove from the oven and set aside to cool before slicing.

TO MAKE THE FRUIT MIXTURE

6. While the cake is baking, in another large bowl, combine the blueberries, strawberries, erythritol–monk fruit blend, and lemon juice. Toss until fully coated and set aside.

TO MAKE THE CHEESECAKE WHIPPED CREAM

7. In a third large bowl, using an electric mixer on high, whip the heavy cream for 3 to 5 minutes, until stiff peaks form, stopping and scraping the bowl once or twice, as needed.

8. In another medium bowl, using an electric mixer on medium high, beat the cream cheese and erythritol–monk fruit blend for 1 to 2 minutes, until smooth and creamy, then stir in the vanilla. Gently fold the whipped cream into the cream cheese mixture until well combined.

9. Assemble the trifle by breaking the slices of the cake into pieces that fit into the bottom of the trifle dish. Add one-third of the berry mixture, followed by one-third of the whipped cream. Alternate the layers two more times, ending with the whipped cream on top.

10. Store leftovers covered in an airtight container for up to 3 days in the refrigerator.

Per serving: Calories: 436; Total Fat: 42g; Total Carbohydrates: 9g; Net Carbs: 7g; Fiber: 2g; Protein: 8g; Sweetener: 22g
Macros: Fat: 84%; Protein: 8%; Carbs: 8%

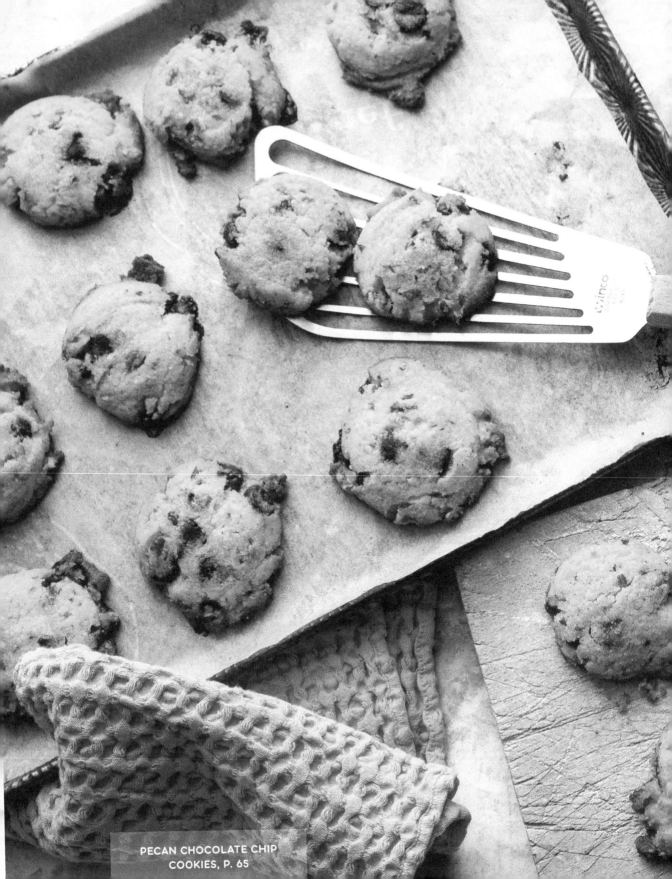

PECAN CHOCOLATE CHIP
COOKIES, P. 65

CHAPTER FIVE

Cookies, Brownies, and Bars

Sugar Cookies 60

Iced Gingerbread Cookies 63

Pecan Chocolate Chip Cookies 65

Carrot Cake Cookies 66

Pistachio Cookies 68

Pumpkin Cookies 70

Salted Peanut Butter Cookies 72

Pumpkin Cheesecake Brownies 73

Blondies 75

Classic Fudgy Brownies 77

Chocolate-Drizzled Pecan Shortbread 78

Macaroon Bars 80

Blueberry Cheesecake Bars 81

Peanut Butter Cake Bars 83

Lemon Bars 84

Sugar Cookies

PREP TIME: 10 minutes **CHILL TIME:** 30 minutes **COOK TIME:** 20 minutes, plus 20 minutes to cool
EQUIPMENT: medium mixing bowl, small mixing bowl, electric mixer, 12-by-17-inch baking sheet, parchment paper, cooling rack, pastry bag (optional)

My family insists on these cookies when we gather. They are reminiscent of the sour cream–based ones many of us grew up on. They have a soft and cake-like texture. If you want something a little less sweet, omit the icing.

FOR THE COOKIES

1 cup granulated erythritol–monk
   fruit blend
8 tablespoons (1 stick) unsalted butter,
   at room temperature
1 teaspoon vanilla extract
2 large eggs, at room temperature
½ cup full-fat sour cream
2½ cups finely milled almond
   flour, sifted

1½ teaspoons baking powder
¼ teaspoon sea salt

FOR THE SOUR CREAM ICING

1¼ cups confectioners' erythritol–monk
   fruit blend
½ cup full-fat sour cream
½ teaspoon vanilla extract

TO MAKE THE COOKIES

1. Preheat the oven to 350°F. Line the baking sheet with parchment paper and set aside.

2. In the medium bowl, using an electric mixer on high, combine the granulated erythritol–monk fruit blend, butter, and vanilla for 1 to 2 minutes, until light and fluffy, stopping and scraping the bowl once or twice, as needed.

3. Add the eggs, one at a time, to the medium bowl, then add the sour cream. Mix until well incorporated. Next add the almond flour, baking powder, and salt and mix until just combined. Put the dough in the refrigerator and chill for 30 minutes.

4. Drop the dough in tablespoons on the prepared baking sheet evenly spaced about 1 inch apart. Bake the cookies for 15 to 20 minutes, until lightly browned around the edges. Transfer the cookies to a cooling rack to fully cool, 15 to 20 minutes.

TO MAKE THE SOUR CREAM ICING

5. In the small bowl, combine the confectioners' erythritol–monk fruit blend, sour cream, and vanilla.

6. Once the cookies are fully cooled, using a spoon or pastry bag, drizzle the icing on top to serve.

7. Store leftovers in the refrigerator for up to 5 days or freeze for up to 3 weeks.

SPICE IT UP: For a more festive look, add a couple drops of food coloring to your icing to match the occasion. Pale pinks, yellows, and blues are gorgeous for Easter, and red and green is perfect for Christmas.

Per serving (2 cookies): Calories: 234; Total Fat: 22g; Total Carbohydrates: 6g; Net Carbs: 4g; Fiber: 2g; Protein: 6g; Sweetener: 36g
Macros: Fat: 82%; Protein: 9%; Carbs: 9%

Iced Gingerbread Cookies

MAKES 24

PREP TIME: 15 minutes **CHILL TIME:** 30 minutes **COOK TIME:** 15 minutes, plus 20 minutes to cool
EQUIPMENT: large mixing bowl, small mixing bowl, electric mixer, 12-by-17-inch baking sheet,
parchment paper, cooling rack, rolling pin, pastry bag (optional), cookie cutter (optional)

This low-carb version of a holiday favorite has a slightly chewy center and crispy edge.
The molasses is technically not keto approved, which is why it's optional here. But if you
can make the molasses work for your macros, it really helps provide that classic gingerbread flavor. If you'd rather not keep molasses around, purchase molasses extract online.

2 cups brown or golden erythritol–monk
  fruit blend; *less sweet: 1¼ cups*

3 large eggs

4 tablespoons (½ stick) unsalted butter,
  at room temperature

1 tablespoon molasses or 1 teaspoon
  molasses extract (optional)

1 teaspoon vanilla extract

4 tablespoons ground cinnamon

3 tablespoons ground ginger

½ teaspoon ground nutmeg

¼ teaspoon ground cloves

3 cups finely milled almond flour

1 tablespoon psyllium husk powder

1½ teaspoons baking powder

¼ teaspoon salt

¼ cup confectioners' erythritol–monk
  fruit blend

1 tablespoon heavy (whipping) cream

1. Preheat the oven to 325°F. Line the baking sheet with parchment paper and set aside.

2. In the large bowl, using an electric mixer on high, beat the brown erythritol–monk
   fruit blend, eggs, butter, molasses (if using), and vanilla until fully incorporated,
   stopping and scraping the bowl once or twice, as needed. Add the cinnamon, ginger,
   nutmeg, and cloves to the mixture and stir to combine.

3. Add the almond flour, psyllium powder, baking powder, and salt and beat on
   medium high until well incorporated.

4. Place the dough between two sheets of parchment paper and flatten with a rolling
   pin. Chill the dough in the refrigerator for 30 minutes.

5. Using a small cookie cutter or small-mouthed glass jar, cut the dough into cookies
   and place them about 1 inch apart, evenly spaced, on the prepared baking sheet.
   Bake for 12 to 15 minutes, until golden brown. Allow them to cool completely on
   the cooling rack, 15 to 20 minutes.

........▶

6. In the small bowl, combine the confectioners' erythritol–monk fruit blend with the heavy cream 1 teaspoon at a time to make the icing. The icing should have a runny consistency. Decorate the cooled cookies using either a pastry bag for fine detail or drizzle the icing on using a fork for a quick, fuss-free decorated cookie.

7. Store leftovers in an airtight container in the refrigerator for up to 5 days or freeze for up to 3 weeks.

SPICE IT UP: If you like your gingerbread cookies on the spicier side, add ¼ teaspoon of black pepper for an extra kick. Or make extra icing and add a few drops of red or green (or both!) food coloring for a more festive look.

Per serving (1 cookie): Calories: 106; Total Fat: 9g; Total Carbohydrates: 5g; Net Carbs: 3g; Fiber: 2g; Protein: 3g; Sweetener: 18g
Macros: Fat: 71%; Protein: 12%; Carbs: 17%

Pecan Chocolate Chip Cookies

PREP TIME: 10 minutes **COOK TIME:** 15 minutes, plus 20 minutes to cool
EQUIPMENT: large mixing bowl, 12-by-17-inch baking sheet, parchment paper, cooling rack

These pecan chocolate chip cookies are soft and chewy. Just smelling them baking in the oven is enough to make me drool.

12 tablespoons (1½ sticks) unsalted butter, at room temperature

½ cup golden or brown erythritol–monk fruit blend

½ cup granulated erythritol–monk fruit blend

1 tablespoon sugar-free maple syrup

2 large eggs

1 tablespoon unflavored gelatin

2 cups finely milled almond flour, sifted

¼ cup coconut flour

2 teaspoons baking powder

¼ teaspoon salt

4 ounces sugar-free chocolate chips

1 cup chopped pecans

1. Preheat the oven to 350°F. Line the baking sheet with parchment paper and set aside.

2. In the large bowl, beat the butter, golden erythritol–monk fruit blend, granulated erythritol–monk fruit blend, and sugar-free maple syrup until light and fluffy. Add the eggs, one at a time, mixing well after each addition. Sprinkle in the gelatin and combine well.

3. Mix in the almond flour, coconut flour, baking powder, and salt. Fold in the sugar-free chocolate chips and pecans.

4. Drop the dough by heaping tablespoons onto the prepared baking sheet, spacing them evenly about 2 inches apart. Flatten the cookies slightly.

5. Bake for 12 to 15 minutes, until golden. Cool on the rack for 15 to 20 minutes before serving.

6. Store leftovers in an airtight container in the refrigerator for up to 5 days or freeze for up to 3 weeks.

Per serving (1 cookie): **Calories:** 253; **Total Fat:** 24g; **Total Carbohydrates:** 6g; **Net Carbs:** 2g; **Fiber:** 4g; **Protein:** 5g; **Sweetener:** 12g
Macros: Fat: 82%; **Protein:** 8%; **Carbs:** 10%

Carrot Cake Cookies

PREP TIME: 10 minutes **CHILL TIME:** 30 minutes **COOK TIME:** 15 minutes, plus 30 minutes to cool
EQUIPMENT: 2 large mixing bowls, medium mixing bowl, electric mixer, baking sheet, cooling rack, small cookie scoop (optional)

These carrot cake cookies are a tasty twist on the classic dessert. Cookies are a great way to build in portion control—plus, they're simpler to make than a whole cake. These cookies are created with coconut flour, which, despite the way it sounds, is not a nut. If you'd like to make them nut-free, simply omit the walnuts.

FOR THE COOKIES

8 tablespoons (1 stick) unsalted butter, at room temperature, plus more for greasing
¾ cup coconut flour
2 teaspoons ground cinnamon
1½ teaspoons baking powder
½ teaspoon ground ginger
¼ teaspoon ground nutmeg
¼ teaspoon salt
¾ cup granulated erythritol–monk fruit blend; *less sweet:* ½ *cup*
4 ounces full-fat cream cheese, at room temperature
½ teaspoon vanilla extract

4 large eggs
¾ cup finely shredded carrots
¼ cup finely chopped walnuts (optional)

FOR THE CREAM CHEESE ICING

1 cup confectioners' erythritol–monk fruit blend
4 tablespoons (½ stick) unsalted butter, at room temperature
2 ounces full-fat cream cheese, at room temperature
3 to 4 tablespoons heavy (whipping) cream
1 teaspoon vanilla extract
¼ teaspoon ground cinnamon

TO MAKE THE COOKIES

1. Preheat the oven to 350°F. Lightly grease the baking sheet with butter and set aside.

2. In a large bowl, combine the coconut flour, cinnamon, baking powder, ginger, nutmeg, and salt and set aside.

3. In another large bowl, using an electric mixer on medium high, beat together the granulated erythritol–monk fruit blend, butter, cream cheese, and vanilla until fully combined, stopping and scraping the bowl once or twice, as needed. Add the eggs, one at a time, mixing well after each addition. Add the dry ingredients to the wet

mixture and beat until fully combined. Fold in the shredded carrots, making sure they're well incorporated into the cookie dough. Fold in the walnuts (if using). Chill the cookie dough for 30 minutes in the refrigerator.

4. Using a cookie scoop or spoon, drop the dough in tablespoon-size cookies onto the prepared baking sheet, evenly spaced and leaving about 1 inch between the cookies. Flatten each ball slightly.

5. Bake for 15 minutes, or until lightly browned around the edges. Allow the cookies to cool on the cooling rack for 30 minutes.

TO MAKE THE CREAM CHEESE ICING

6. In the medium bowl, using an electric mixer on high, mix the confectioners' erythritol–monk fruit blend, butter, and cream cheese for 1 to 2 minutes until smooth, stopping and scraping the bowl once or twice, as needed. Add 3 tablespoons of heavy cream, the vanilla, and cinnamon and mix well. Add the additional 1 tablespoon of cream to thin the icing, if necessary.

7. Using a fork, drizzle the cooled cookies with icing before serving.

8. Store leftovers in an airtight container in the refrigerator for up to 5 days or freeze for up to 3 weeks.

INGREDIENT TIP: The carrots should be freshly grated using the fine holes of a box grater or a food processor. The pre-shredded carrots won't work. Once grated, squeeze the carrots dry with a paper towel to remove excess moisture.

Per serving (2 cookies): Calories: 213; Total Fat: 21g; Total Carbohydrates: 3g; Net Carbs: 2g; Fiber: 1g; Protein: 3g; Sweetener: 28g
Macros: Fat: 88%; Protein: 7%; Carbs: 5%

Pistachio Cookies

PREP TIME: 10 minutes **CHILL TIME:** 30 minutes **COOK TIME:** 20 minutes, plus 30 minutes to cool
EQUIPMENT: medium mixing bowl, large mixing bowl, small mixing bowl, electric mixer, 12-by-17-inch baking sheet, small cookie scoop (optional), parchment paper, cooling rack

These chewy, cream cheese–based pistachio cookies nail the salty-sweet combo. If you'd prefer a less sweet option, omit the icing. For a festive look, add a couple drops of green food coloring to the cookies.

FOR THE COOKIES

1 cup coconut flour

1½ teaspoons baking powder

¼ teaspoon salt

1 cup granulated erythritol–monk fruit blend; *less sweet: ¾ cup*

8 tablespoons (1 stick) unsalted butter, at room temperature

4 ounces full-fat cream cheese, at room temperature

1 teaspoon vanilla extract

4 large eggs, at room temperature

¼ cup finely chopped pistachios, plus more for garnish

FOR THE VANILLA ICING

½ cup confectioners' erythritol–monk fruit blend

3 tablespoons heavy (whipping) cream

1 teaspoon vanilla extract

TO MAKE THE COOKIES

1. Preheat the oven to 350°F. Line the baking sheet with parchment paper and set aside.

2. In the medium bowl, stir together the coconut flour, baking powder, and salt and set aside.

3. In the large bowl, using an electric mixer on medium, beat together the granulated erythritol–monk fruit blend, butter, cream cheese, and vanilla until fully combined, stopping and scraping the bowl once or twice, as needed. Add the eggs, one at a time, mixing well after each addition. Add the dry ingredients to the wet mixture, stirring until fully combined. Stir in the pistachios and chill the dough for at least 30 minutes in the refrigerator.

4. Using a cookie scoop or spoon, drop the dough in tablespoon-size cookies onto the prepared baking sheet, evenly spaced, leaving about 1 inch between the cookies. Flatten each ball slightly.

5. Bake for 15 to 18 minutes, or until lightly browned around the edges. Cool on the rack for 30 minutes.

TO MAKE THE VANILLA ICING

6. In the small bowl, combine the confectioners' erythritol–monk fruit blend, heavy cream, and vanilla.

7. Using a fork, drizzle the icing on top of the cooled cookies and top with chopped pistachios before serving.

8. Store the cookies in an airtight container in the refrigerator for up to 5 days or freeze for up to 3 weeks.

VARIATION TIP: Change up the flavor by swapping the pistachios for almonds and adding ½ teaspoon of almond extract to make almond cookies instead.

Per serving (3 cookies): Calories: 272; Total Fat: 27g; Total Carbohydrates: 4g; Net Carbs: 3g; Fiber: 1g; Protein: 5g; Sweetener: 36g
Macros: Fat: 86%; Protein: 8%; Carbs: 6%

Pumpkin Cookies

PREP TIME: 10 minutes **CHILL TIME:** 1 hour **COOK TIME:** 25 minutes, plus 30 minutes to cool
EQUIPMENT: medium mixing bowl, large mixing bowl, small mixing bowl, electric mixer, 12-by-17-inch baking sheet, small cookie scoop (optional), parchment paper, cooling rack, pastry bag

If you're a pumpkin fan, you're going to love these perfectly spiced and incredibly soft cake-like cookies. Enjoy them with your favorite hot tea to get that comfy fall feeling any time of the year.

FOR THE COOKIES

¾ cup coconut flour

1½ teaspoons baking powder

1 teaspoon ground cinnamon

½ teaspoon ground ginger

¼ teaspoon ground nutmeg

¼ teaspoon salt

¾ cup granulated erythritol–monk fruit blend; *less sweet: ½ cup*

8 tablespoons (1 stick) unsalted butter, at room temperature

4 ounces full-fat cream cheese, room temperature

½ teaspoon vanilla extract

4 large eggs, at room temperature

½ cup canned pumpkin puree

FOR THE ICING

½ cup confectioners' erythritol–monk fruit blend

4 to 5 tablespoons heavy (whipping) cream, divided

TO MAKE THE COOKIES

1. Preheat the oven to 350°F. Line the baking sheet with parchment paper and set aside.

2. In the medium bowl, combine the coconut flour, baking powder, cinnamon, ginger, nutmeg, and salt and set aside.

3. In the large bowl, using an electric mixer on high, beat together the granulated erythritol–monk fruit blend, butter, cream cheese, and vanilla until fully combined, stopping and scraping the bowl once or twice, as needed. Add the eggs, one at a time, mixing well after each addition, then stir in the pumpkin puree and continue to mix. Add the dry ingredients to the wet mixture and mix on low until combined.

4. Chill the cookie dough for 45 minutes to 1 hour.

5. Using a cookie scoop or spoon, drop the dough in tablespoon-size cookies onto the prepared baking sheet, evenly spaced, and leaving about 1 inch between the cookies. Flatten each ball slightly.

6. Bake for 20 to 25 minutes, or until lightly browned around the edges. Remove the cookies from the oven and let them cool on the rack for 30 minutes.

TO MAKE THE ICING

7. While the cookies bake, in a small bowl, combine the confectioners' erythritol–monk fruit blend with 2 tablespoons of heavy cream, adding 1 tablespoon more at a time, if needed. The icing should be runny enough to easily drizzle.

8. Using a pastry bag or fork, drizzle the cookies with the icing. Let the icing set on the cookies for about 10 minutes before eating.

9. Store the cookies in an airtight container in the refrigerator for up to 5 days or freeze for up to 3 weeks.

VARIATION TIP: Add ¼ teaspoon of orange extract to the icing for a tangy, citrusy kick. You'll be surprised at how well the orange icing complements the autumnal flavors of the pumpkin cookie!

Per serving (2 cookies): Calories: 246; Total Fat: 24g; Total Carbohydrates: 4g; Net Carbs: 3g; Fiber: 1g; Protein: 5g; Sweetener: 30g
Macros: Fat: 86%; Protein: 8%; Carbs: 6%

Salted Peanut Butter Cookies

PREP TIME: 10 minutes **COOK TIME:** 40 minutes
EQUIPMENT: large mixing bowl, electric mixer, 12-by-17-inch baking sheet, small cookie scoop
(optional), parchment paper

These slightly chewy cookies are elevated by the addition of sea salt flakes. It's hard to believe they are made with only gluten-free, low-carb ingredients, but thankfully they are. Make them dairy-free by swapping out the softened butter for solid coconut oil.

1 cup all-natural peanut butter
  (no added sugar)
1 cup granulated erythritol–monk fruit
  blend; *less sweet: ½ cup*
8 tablespoons (1 stick) unsalted butter,
  at room temperature

1 large egg, at room temperature
1 cup finely milled almond flour
1 teaspoon baking powder
½ teaspoon sea salt

1. Preheat the oven to 350°F. Line the baking sheet with parchment paper.

2. In the large bowl, using an electric mixer on medium high, combine the peanut butter, erythritol–monk fruit blend, butter, and egg and mix until combined, stopping and scraping the bowl once or twice, as needed. Add the almond flour and baking powder. Mix on low until fully incorporated.

3. Using a small cookie scoop or spoon, place tablespoon-size cookies on the prepared baking sheet and flatten them with the tines of a fork to make a crisscross design. Sprinkle the tops with the salt. Bake for 10 to 12 minutes, until lightly browned around the edges.

4. Allow the cookies to cool completely before eating.

5. Carefully handle these cookies when storing because they can be very fragile. They will last in the refrigerator for up to 5 days or in the freezer for up to 3 weeks.

INGREDIENT TIP: Using a natural, sugar-free peanut butter is very important for your macros and will impact the overall sweetness of these cookies.

Per serving (3 cookies): **Calories:** 360; **Total Fat:** 32g; **Total Carbohydrates:** 3g; **Net Carbs:** 1g; **Fiber:** 2g;
Protein: 11g; **Sweetener:** 24g
Macros: Fat: 82%; **Protein:** 14%; **Carbs:** 4%

Pumpkin Cheesecake Brownies

PREP TIME: 15 minutes **COOK TIME:** 25 minutes, plus 15 minutes to cool **CHILL TIME:** 35 minutes
EQUIPMENT: 2 medium mixing bowls, electric mixer, 8-by-8-inch baking pan, small microwave-safe bowl, parchment paper, cooling rack

What to do when you can't decide between a brownie or pumpkin pie? You mix up a batch of pumpkin cheesecake brownies! These treats will satisfy any pumpkin spice cravings.

FOR THE BROWNIES

12 tablespoons (1½ sticks) unsalted butter, at room temperature, plus more for greasing

4 ounces unsweetened baking chocolate, coarsely chopped

1¼ cups granulated erythritol–monk fruit blend; *less sweet: 1 cup*

3 large eggs, at room temperature

1 teaspoon vanilla extract

1 cup finely milled almond flour, sifted

1 teaspoon baking powder

¼ teaspoon sea salt

FOR THE PUMPKIN CHEESECAKE SWIRL

8 ounces full-fat cream cheese, at room temperature

½ cup canned pumpkin puree

¼ cup granulated erythritol–monk fruit blend

1 large egg, at room temperature

1 teaspoon vanilla extract

1 teaspoon ground cinnamon

½ teaspoon ground ginger

¼ teaspoon ground nutmeg

¼ teaspoon ground allspice

TO MAKE THE BROWNIES

1. Preheat the oven to 350°F. Line the bottom of the baking pan with parchment paper and grease the sides of the pan with butter.

2. In the small microwave-safe bowl, melt the chocolate and butter together in the microwave, in 30-second intervals, until fully melted. Stir well and allow to cool for 5 minutes.

3. In a medium bowl, using an electric mixer on low, whisk the chocolate mixture and erythritol–monk fruit blend until fully combined. With the mixer on medium high, add the eggs, one at a time, until well combined, stopping and scraping the bowl once or twice, as needed. Mix in the vanilla until the batter is smooth and the sweetener has fully dissolved.

4. Stir in the almond flour, baking powder, and salt until fully blended, being careful not to overmix. Spread two-thirds of the batter into the bottom of the baking pan and set aside.

TO MAKE THE PUMPKIN CHEESECAKE SWIRL

5. In another medium bowl, using an electric mixer on medium high, combine the cream cheese, pumpkin puree, erythritol–monk fruit blend, egg, vanilla, cinnamon, ginger, nutmeg, and allspice and mix, stopping and scraping the bowl once or twice, as needed, until well combined. Pour the cheesecake swirl on the top of the brownie batter. Then add the remainder of the brownie mix, by spoonfuls, on top of the cheesecake layer. Using a knife, gently swirl the two batters together.

6. Bake for 20 to 25 minutes, or until the center is just set but still jiggles. Check for this consistency at the 20-minute mark and add more time if needed.

7. Allow the brownies to fully cool on the rack, about 15 minutes. Refrigerate the cooled brownies and allow them to further set for 30 to 35 minutes before slicing into 16 squares before serving.

8. Store leftovers in an airtight container in the refrigerator for up to 5 days or freeze for up to 3 weeks.

VARIATION TIP: The cheesecake swirl is totally customizable! Omit the pumpkin puree and spices, and use 1 teaspoon of mint or hazelnut extract for a different flavored brownie.

Per serving (1 brownie): Calories: 228; Total Fat: 21g; Total Carbohydrates: 5g; Net Carbs: 3g; Fiber: 2g; Protein: 5g; Sweetener: 18g
Macros: Fat: 83%; Protein: 9%; Carbs: 8%

Blondies

PREP TIME: 10 minutes **COOK TIME:** 35 minutes
EQUIPMENT: large mixing bowl, electric mixer, 8-by-8-inch baking pan

These soft and chewy blondies have a buttery crumb. You won't miss the molasses flavor in traditional blondies thanks to the brown erythritol–monk fruit blend. Feel free to throw in a handful of chopped walnuts or sugar-free chocolate chips.

4 tablespoons (½ stick) unsalted butter, at room temperature, plus more for greasing

1 cup brown or golden erythritol–monk fruit blend; *less sweet:* ½ *cup*

4 ounces full-fat cream cheese, at room temperature

1 teaspoon vanilla extract

2 large eggs

½ cup finely milled almond flour

2½ tablespoons coconut flour

1 teaspoon baking powder

¼ teaspoon xanthan gum (optional)

⅛ teaspoon sea salt

1. Preheat the oven to 350°F. Grease the baking pan with butter and set aside.

2. In the large bowl, using an electric mixer on medium high, beat together the brown erythritol–monk fruit blend, cream cheese, butter, and vanilla until combined. Add the eggs, one at a time, mixing well after each addition, stopping and scraping the bowl once or twice, as needed. Fold in the almond flour, coconut flour, baking powder, xanthan gum (if using), and salt. Spread the batter evenly into the prepared baking pan.

3. Bake for 30 to 35 minutes, or until golden brown. Allow the blondies to cool completely before slicing into 24 bars and serving.

4. Store leftovers in an airtight container in the refrigerator for 5 days or freeze for up to 3 weeks

INGREDIENT TIP: Adding the xanthan gum is optional, but it's what makes these blondies a little chewy, like the carb-filled version.

Per serving (1 blondie): Calories: 53; Total Fat: 5g; Total Carbohydrates: 1g; Net Carbs: 1g; Fiber: 0g; Protein: 2g; Sweetener: 8g
Macros: Fat: 84%; Protein: 10%; Carbs: 6%

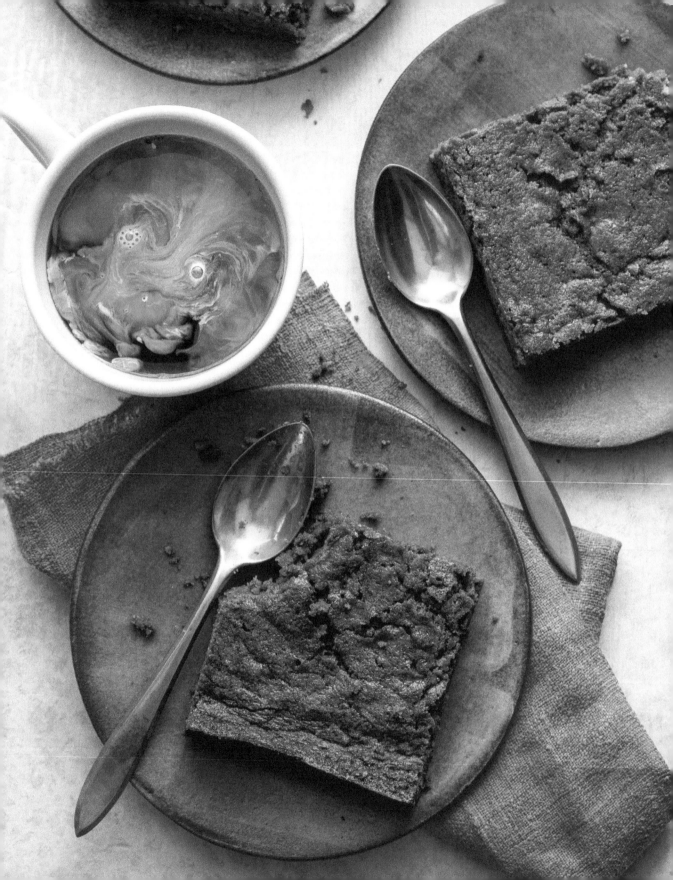

Classic Fudgy Brownies

PREP TIME: 10 minutes **COOK TIME:** 25 minutes, plus 15 minutes to cool **CHILL TIME:** 35 minutes
EQUIPMENT: medium mixing bowl, electric mixer, 8-by-8-inch baking pan, small microwave-safe bowl, parchment paper, cooling rack

These moist keto-friendly brownies will have you jumping for joy. Make sure you don't overbake them!

4 ounces unsweetened baking chocolate, coarsely chopped

12 tablespoons (1½ sticks) unsalted butter, at room temperature

1¼ cups granulated erythritol–monk fruit blend; *less sweet: 1 cup*

3 large eggs, at room temperature

1 teaspoon vanilla extract

1 cup finely milled almond flour, sifted

1 teaspoon baking powder

¼ teaspoon sea salt

1. Preheat the oven to 350°F. Line the bottom of the baking pan with parchment paper.

2. In the small microwave-safe bowl, melt the chocolate and butter together in the microwave, in 30-second intervals, until fully melted. Stir well and cool for 5 minutes.

3. In the medium bowl, whisk together the erythritol–monk fruit blend and chocolate mixture. Using an electric mixer on medium high, mix in the eggs, one at a time, until well combined. Mix in the vanilla until the batter is smooth.

4. Whisk in the almond flour, baking powder, and salt, taking care not to overmix or the brownies will be cakey. Spread the batter into the baking pan.

5. Bake for 20 to 25 minutes, or until the center is just set but still jiggles. Check for this consistency at the 20-minute mark and add more time if needed.

6. Allow to fully cool on the rack, about 15 minutes. Refrigerate the cooled brownies, allowing them to set for 30 to 35 minutes before cutting and serving.

7. Store leftovers in an airtight container in the refrigerator for up to 5 days or freeze for up to 3 weeks.

Per serving (1 brownie): Calories: 171; Total Fat: 16g; Total Carbohydrates: 3g; Net Carbs: 1g; Fiber: 2g; Protein: 4g; Sweetener: 15g
Macros: Fat: 84%; Protein: 9%; Carbs: 7%

Chocolate-Drizzled Pecan Shortbread

MAKES 24 BARS

PREP TIME: 10 minutes **CHILL TIME:** 45 minutes **COOK TIME:** 40 minutes
EQUIPMENT: medium mixing bowl, 9-by-9-inch baking pan, microwave-safe bowl, pastry bag (optional)

Crunchy pecans and a chocolate drizzle make these bars an irresistible, over-the-top version of the classic shortbread. To get the best results, make these cookies by hand and not with a food processor. Yes, it takes a bit more effort, but I promise it's worth it.

FOR THE SHORTBREAD

2½ cups finely milled almond
    flour, sifted
¾ cup granulated erythritol–monk
    fruit blend
½ cup finely chopped pecans
1 teaspoon baking powder
½ teaspoon sea salt

1 cup (2 sticks) unsalted butter, chilled
    and thinly sliced
1½ teaspoons vanilla extract

FOR THE CHOCOLATE DRIZZLE

5 ounces sugar-free dark chocolate chips
1 teaspoon coconut oil

TO MAKE THE SHORTBREAD

1. Preheat the oven to 300°F.

2. In the medium bowl, whisk together the almond flour, erythritol–monk fruit blend, pecans, baking powder, and salt. Add the butter and vanilla to the flour mixture. Using your fingers, rub the pieces of butter into the flour mixture, working the mixture for about 5 minutes until the dough comes together.

3. Press the dough into the baking pan and chill in the refrigerator for at least 45 minutes.

4. Using a fork, make a few indents with the tines on top of the shortbread to create that classic shortbread look.

5. Bake for 35 to 40 minutes, or until the edges are lightly golden brown. Remove and let cool in the pan completely before slicing into 24 bars.

TO MAKE THE CHOCOLATE DRIZZLE

6. In the small microwave-safe bowl, melt the chocolate and coconut oil together in the microwave in 30-second intervals. Using a fork or a pastry bag, drizzle the cooled bars with melted chocolate. Allow the chocolate to set before serving.

7. Store leftovers in an airtight container for up to 5 days in the refrigerator or in the freezer for up to 3 weeks.

KEEP IN MIND: It's important not to skip the step of placing the unbaked bars in the refrigerator to chill before baking—chilling will ensure they have the traditional crisp texture of shortbread.

Per serving (2 bars): Calories: 331; Total Fat: 32g; Total Carbohydrates: 8g; Net Carbs: 4g; Fiber: 4g; Protein: 6g; Sweetener: 12g
Macros: Fat: 84%; Protein: 7%; Carbs: 9%

Macaroon Bars

PREP TIME: 10 minutes **COOK TIME:** 35 minutes, plus 20 minutes to cool
EQUIPMENT: large mixing bowl, spatula, electric mixer, 8-by-8-inch baking pan

These bars have a chewy center and slightly crisp exterior that makes them irresistible. When working with the beaten egg whites, take care to maintain their delightfully airy texture. And don't toss those egg yolks! Use them to make Chocolate Pudding (page 44).

Coconut oil, for greasing

4 large egg whites

½ teaspoon cream of tartar

3 cups unsweetened shredded coconut

1 cup granulated erythritol–monk fruit blend; *less sweet: ¾ cup*

1 teaspoon almond extract

1. Preheat the oven to 350°F. Grease the baking pan with coconut oil and set aside.

2. In the large bowl, using an electric mixer on high, beat the egg whites and cream of tartar for 3 to 5 minutes, until medium-stiff peaks form. Using a spatula, gently fold in the coconut, erythritol–monk fruit blend, and almond extract. Spread evenly into the prepared baking pan.

3. Bake for 30 to 35 minutes, or until lightly browned. Allow to cool 15 to 20 minutes before slicing into 18 bars and serving.

4. Store leftovers in an airtight container in the refrigerator for up to 5 days or freeze for up to 3 weeks.

SPICE IT UP: For chocolate lovers, either dip these macaroon bars in melted chocolate, or drizzle the chocolate over them. Simply melt 5 ounces of sugar-free chocolate chips and 1 teaspoon of coconut oil in a microwave-safe bowl in the microwave in 30-second intervals.

Per serving (2 bars): **Calories:** 107; **Total Fat:** 9g; **Total Carbohydrates:** 4g; **Net Carbs:** 2g; **Fiber:** 2g; **Protein:** 2g; **Sweetener:** 21g
Macros: Fat: 74%; **Protein:** 9%; **Carbs:** 17%

Blueberry Cheesecake Bars

MAKES 12

PREP TIME: 10 minutes **COOK TIME:** 50 minutes, plus 50 minutes to cool **CHILL TIME:** 3 hours
EQUIPMENT: medium mixing bowl, large mixing bowl, electric mixer, 8-by-8-inch baking pan,
aluminum foil, cooling rack

With these bars, you can enjoy all the flavor of regular cheesecake in a convenient,
portion-controlled treat. To make them less carby, decrease or eliminate the berries.

FOR THE CRUST

1½ cups finely milled almond flour

5 tablespoons unsalted butter, melted

2 tablespoons granulated erythritol–
monk fruit blend

⅛ teaspoon salt

FOR THE CHEESECAKE

16 ounces full-fat cream cheese, at room
temperature

⅔ cup granulated erythritol–monk fruit
blend; *less sweet:* ⅓ *cup*

2 large eggs

2 teaspoons grated lemon zest

1 tablespoon freshly squeezed
lemon juice

1 teaspoon vanilla extract

2 cups frozen blueberries, unthawed

TO MAKE THE CRUST

1. Preheat the oven to 350°F. Line the baking pan with aluminum foil, leaving enough
to hang over the sides.

2. In the medium bowl, combine the almond flour, butter, erythritol–monk fruit
blend, and salt. Press the mixture into the prepared pan and bake for 12 to
15 minutes, until lightly browned. Set aside and allow to completely cool, about
20 minutes. Leave the oven on.

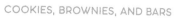

TO MAKE THE CHEESECAKE

3. In the large bowl, using an electric mixer on medium, beat the cream cheese for 1 minute, until smooth. Add the erythritol–monk fruit blend, eggs, lemon zest, lemon juice, and vanilla and beat together for about 3 minutes, stopping and scraping the bowl once or twice, as needed, until smooth and creamy. Gently fold in the blueberries. Spoon the batter into the cooled crust and spread evenly.

4. Bake for 30 to 35 minutes at 350°F, or until the cheesecake has set and the edges are lightly browned. The bars will be a little puffy but will sink slightly down as they cool. Cool for 30 minutes at room temperature on the rack, then chill in the refrigerator for at least 3 hours. Using the aluminum foil overhang, lift the cheesecake out of the pan and cut into 12 bars before serving.

5. Store leftovers in an airtight container in the refrigerator for up to 5 days or in the freezer for up to 3 weeks.

VARIATION TIP: You can easily swap out the blueberries for any other berry or even do a mixed berry option!

Per serving (1 bar) : Calories: 268; Total Fat: 25g; Total Carbohydrates: 8g; Net Carbs: 6g; Fiber: 2g; Protein: 6g; Sweetener: 13g
Macros: Fat: 80%; Protein: 9%; Carbs: 11%;

Peanut Butter Cake Bars

MAKES 24

PREP TIME: 10 minutes **COOK TIME:** 45 minutes, plus 20 minutes to cool
EQUIPMENT: large mixing bowl, electric mixer, 9-by-13-inch baking sheet, cooling rack, small microwave-safe bowl, toothpicks

These bars may convert peanut butter fans into ketoers. To achieve a salty-sweet flavor, top the bars with ½ cup of peanuts and a sprinkling of flaky sea salt.

12 tablespoons (1½ sticks) unsalted butter, at room temperature, plus more for greasing

2 cups granulated erythritol–monk fruit blend; *less sweet: 1½ cups*

8 ounces full-fat cream cheese, at room temperature

1 teaspoon vanilla extract

2¼ cups all-natural peanut butter (no added sugar), divided

½ cup sour cream

5 large eggs, at room temperature

2 cups finely milled almond flour

1 cup whey protein or an additional 1 cup almond flour

2 teaspoons baking powder

¼ teaspoon salt

1. Preheat the oven to 350°F. Grease the baking sheet with butter and set aside.

2. In the large bowl, using an electric mixer on medium high, cream the erythritol–monk fruit blend, cream cheese, butter, and vanilla for 2 to 3 minutes, stopping and scraping the bowl once or twice, as needed, until light and fluffy. Add half the peanut butter and sour cream. Add the eggs, one at a time, until fully incorporated. Stir in the almond flour, whey protein, baking powder, and salt. Spread evenly into the prepared pan.

3. Bake for 40 to 45 minutes, or until a toothpick inserted into the center comes out clean. Cool on the rack for 20 minutes.

4. While the bars are cooling, in a microwave-safe bowl, melt the remaining peanut butter in the microwave in 20-second intervals. Drizzle on top of the bars and allow to set for 10 minutes before slicing into 24 bars to serve. Store leftovers in an airtight container in the refrigerator for up to 5 days or freeze for up to 3 weeks.

Per serving (2 bars): Calories: 638; Total Fat: 53g; Total Carbohydrates: 8g; Net Carbs: 5g; Fiber: 3g; Protein: 26g; Sweetener: 32g
Macros: Fat: 75%; Protein: 16%; Carbs: 9%

Lemon Bars

PREP TIME: 10 minutes COOK TIME: 1 hour CHILL TIME: 2 hours
EQUIPMENT: 2 medium mixing bowls, 8-by-8-inch baking pan, parchment paper

A tart lemon curd filling and a shortbread crust make these bars a tangy treat. Light and refreshing, they are perfect when you want just a little something sweet after dinner, or really any time of the day.

FOR THE CRUST

1 cup (2 sticks) unsalted butter, melted
⅓ cup granulated erythritol–monk
   fruit blend
1 teaspoon vanilla extract
½ teaspoon salt
2 cups finely milled almond flour, sifted
1 tablespoon coconut flour

FOR THE FILLING

9 large egg yolks
1 cup granulated erythritol–monk
   fruit blend
2 teaspoons grated lemon zest
⅛ teaspoon salt
¾ cup freshly squeezed lemon juice
Confectioners' erythritol–monk fruit
   blend, for dusting (optional)

TO MAKE THE CRUST

1. Preheat the oven to 325°F. Line the baking pan with parchment paper, leaving enough to hang over the sides.

2. In a medium bowl, combine the melted butter, granulated erythritol–monk fruit blend, vanilla, and salt. Stir in the almond flour and coconut flour to combine. Press the mixture into the prepared pan and bake for 25 to 30 minutes, until the edges are slightly browned. Leave the oven on.

TO MAKE THE FILLING

3. While the crust bakes, in another medium bowl, whisk the egg yolks, granulated erythritol–monk fruit blend, lemon zest, and salt until well combined. Slowly pour in the lemon juice and continue to whisk until it is well incorporated.

4. Pour the filling into the warm crust and spread evenly.

5. Bake for 25 to 30 minutes, until the center is mostly set but has a little jiggle. Allow the filling to cool completely at room temperature, 15 to 20 minutes. Refrigerate for 1 to 1½ hours until chilled. Lift out of the pan using the overhanging parchment paper and cut into 12 bars. Serve chilled and dusted with confectioners' erythritol–monk fruit blend (if using).

6. Store leftovers in an airtight container in the refrigerator for up to 5 days or in the freezer, individually wrapped, and put in a freezer bag for up to 3 weeks.

VARIATION TIP: Change it up by adding lime juice and zest as well as lemon to make these into lemon-lime bars. I recommend using ¼ cup of lime juice with ½ cup of lemon juice and 1 teaspoon each of lemon and lime zest.

Per serving: Calories: 286; Total Fat: 27g; Total Carbohydrates: 6g; Net Carbs: 4g; Fiber: 2g; Protein: 6g; Sweetener: 21g
Macros: Fat: 85%; Protein: 8%; Carbs: 7%

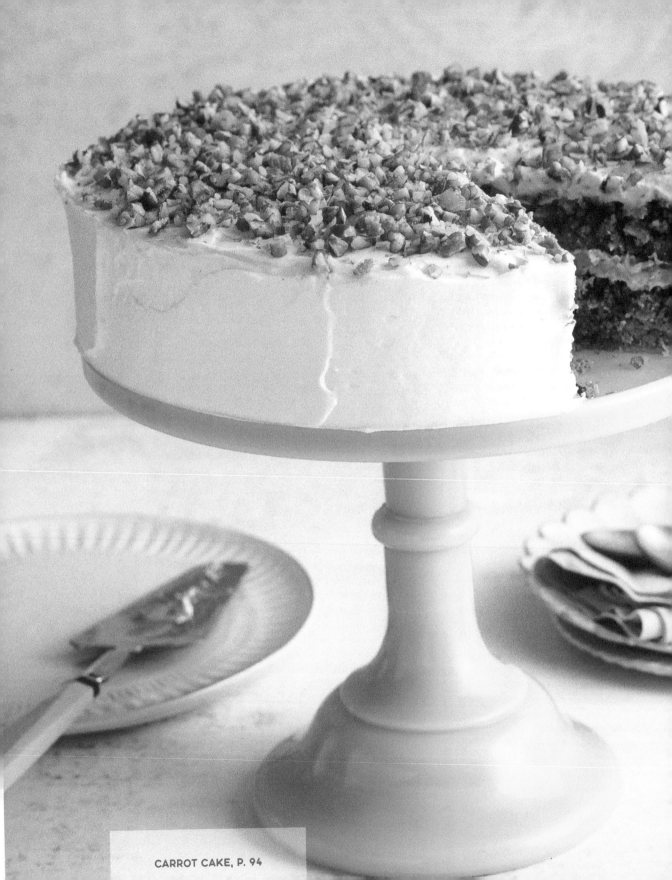

CARROT CAKE, P. 94

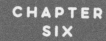

CHAPTER SIX

Cakes and Breads

Brown Butter Bundt Cake 88

Chocolate Sheet Cake 90

Toasted Coconut Cake 92

Carrot Cake 94

Salted Caramel Cupcakes 97

Tiramisu 99

No-Bake Chocolate Raspberry Cheesecake 101

Mini Cranberry Cheesecakes 103

Classic Cheesecake 105

Nut-Free Pumpkin Bread 108

Chocolate Chip Scones 109

Strawberry Rhubarb Scones 111

Blueberry Muffins 113

Dairy-Free Cranberry Muffins 115

Dairy-Free Chocolate Donuts 116

Poppy Seed Pound Cake 118

Brown Butter Bundt Cake

SERVES 14

PREP TIME: 10 minutes **CHILL TIME:** 2 hours 20 minutes
COOK TIME: 1 hour, plus 40 minutes to cool and 10 minutes to set
EQUIPMENT: 2 large mixing bowls, small mixing bowl, electric mixer, 2 small saucepans, 12-cup bundt pan, cooling rack, toothpicks

This moist pound cake gets its nutty flavor from browned butter. It goes well with a delicious cup of coffee or afternoon tea. For extra flair, top the cake with lightly toasted sliced almonds immediately after you apply the icing.

FOR THE CAKE

12 tablespoons (1½ sticks) unsalted
   butter, at room temperature, plus more
   for greasing
2½ cups finely milled almond
   flour, sifted
1 cup coconut flour
2 teaspoons baking powder
¼ teaspoon sea salt
½ cup heavy (whipping) cream
¼ teaspoon distilled white vinegar
8 ounces full-fat cream cheese, at room
   temperature

1¼ cups granulated erythritol–monk
   fruit blend
1 teaspoon vanilla extract
5 large eggs, at room temperature

FOR THE ICING

4 tablespoons (½ stick) unsalted butter,
   at room temperature
¾ cup confectioners' erythritol–monk
   fruit blend
¼ cup heavy (whipping) cream
¼ teaspoon sea salt

TO MAKE THE CAKE

1. Preheat the oven to 350°F. Grease the bundt pan with butter and set aside.

2. In a small saucepan, brown the butter over medium heat, stirring constantly. Once the butter begins to foam and bubble, after 2 to 4 minutes, you should begin to see browned bits on the bottom of the pan. At this point, remove the pan from the heat immediately and continue to stir until the butter turns to a golden amber color. Transfer the browned butter to the refrigerator for about 2 hours to allow the butter to become opaque and solid. Remove the pan from the refrigerator and allow the browned butter to come to room temperature and soften slightly, about 20 minutes.

3. In a large bowl, combine the almond flour, coconut flour, baking powder, and salt.

4. In the small bowl, mix the heavy cream and vinegar and set aside.

5. In another large bowl, using an electric mixer on medium high, beat the cream cheese and granulated erythritol–monk fruit blend for 2 to 3 minutes, until light fluffy. Add the browned butter and beat until well incorporated. Add the vanilla and the eggs, one at a time, mixing well after each addition, stopping and scraping the bowl once or twice, as needed. Slowly add all the dry ingredients, 1 tablespoon at a time while continuing to mix. Fold in the heavy cream and vinegar mixture.

6. Pour the batter into the prepared bundt pan and bake in the center rack for 45 to 50 minutes, until a toothpick inserted halfway between the tube and the edge comes out clean. Allow the cake to cool in the pan for 10 minutes before inverting and transferring to the cooling rack for 15 to 20 minutes.

TO MAKE THE ICING

7. In another small saucepan, brown the butter over medium heat, stirring constantly. Once the butter begins to foam and bubble, after 2 to 4 minutes, you should begin to see browned bits on the bottom of the pan. At this point, remove from the heat immediately and continue to stir until the butter turns to a golden amber color. Add the confectioners' erythritol–monk fruit blend, heavy cream, and salt and stir until well combined.

8. While the icing is still warm, drizzle it over the top of the cake allowing it to seep into the cake. Let set for another 10 minutes before slicing into 14 wedges and serving.

9. Store leftovers in an airtight container in the refrigerator for up to 5 days or freeze for up to 3 weeks.

Per serving: Calories: 381; Total Fat: 37g; Total Carbohydrates: 7g; Net Carbs: 4g; Fiber: 3g; Protein: 8g; Sweetener: 27g
Macros: Fat: 85%; Protein: 8%; Carbs: 7%

Chocolate Sheet Cake

SERVES 18

PREP TIME: 10 minutes **COOK TIME:** 50 minutes, plus 20 minutes to cool
EQUIPMENT: 2 medium mixing bowls, large mixing bowl, electric mixer, microwave-safe bowl,
9-by-13-inch baking sheet, toothpicks

This velvety chocolate sheet cake is topped with a luscious chocolate buttercream frosting. It's large enough to feed a crowd, which makes it perfect for birthdays, holidays, or any special occasion.

FOR THE CAKE

8 tablespoons (1 stick) unsalted butter, at room temperature, plus more for greasing

2 ounces unsweetened baking chocolate, coarsely chopped

1¼ cups coconut flour

¼ cup dark cocoa powder

3½ teaspoons baking powder

½ teaspoon baking soda

½ teaspoon sea salt

1½ cups granulated erythritol–monk fruit blend

8 ounces full-fat cream cheese, at room temperature

2 teaspoons vanilla extract

8 large eggs, at room temperature

½ cup full-fat sour cream

FOR THE FROSTING

1 cup (2 sticks) unsalted butter, at room temperature

2 ounces full-fat cream cheese, at room temperature

2 cups confectioners' erythritol–monk fruit blend

⅔ cup unsweetened natural cocoa powder

⅔ cup heavy (whipping) cream

1 teaspoon vanilla extract

¼ teaspoon sea salt

TO MAKE THE CAKE

1. Preheat the oven to 350°F. Grease the baking sheet with butter and set aside.

2. In the small microwave-safe bowl, melt the baking chocolate in the microwave in 30-second intervals and set aside.

3. In a medium bowl, combine the coconut flour, dark cocoa powder, baking powder, baking soda, and salt.

4. In the large bowl, using an electric mixer on medium high, beat together the granulated erythritol–monk fruit blend, cream cheese, butter, and vanilla for 2 to 3 minutes, until light and fluffy. Add the melted chocolate and the eggs, one at a time, mixing well after each addition, stopping and scraping the bowl as needed. Slowly add the dry ingredients while mixing on low, scraping down the sides of the bowl.

5. Gently fold the sour cream into the cake batter until fully incorporated, but be careful not to overmix. Spread the cake batter in the prepared cake pan.

6. Bake the cake for 45 to 50 minutes, until a toothpick inserted into the center comes out clean or with only a tiny bit of crumb. Check at the 35-minute mark. Cool fully in the pan, about 20 minutes.

TO MAKE THE FROSTING

7. While the cake is baking, in another medium bowl, using an electric mixer on high, cream the butter and cream cheese. Add 1 cup of confectioners' erythritol–monk fruit blend, ⅓ cup of cocoa powder, and ⅓ cup of heavy cream and continue to beat on high, stopping and scraping the bowl once or twice, as needed, until fully combined. Add the remaining 1 cup of confectioners' erythritol–monk fruit blend and ⅓ cup of cocoa powder and combine well at high speed until well mixed. Add the remaining ⅓ cup of heavy cream, the vanilla, and salt and mix until fully incorporated.

8. Wait until the cake has cooled completely before frosting. Cut into 18 pieces and serve. Store leftovers in an airtight container in the refrigerator for up to 5 days.

KEEP IN MIND: The butter and cream cheese mixture in step 4 will not fully combine until you add the dry ingredients.

Per serving: Calories: 328; Total Fat: 33g; Total Carbohydrates: 6g; Net Carbs: 3g; Fiber: 3g; Protein: 6g; Sweetener: 37g
Macros: Fat: 88%; Protein: 7%; Carbs: 5%

Toasted Coconut Cake

SERVES 12

PREP TIME: 10 minutes COOK TIME: 45 minutes, plus 25 minutes to cool
EQUIPMENT: medium mixing bowl, small mixing bowl, 12-by-17-inch baking sheet, 9-inch round cake pan, parchment paper, toothpicks

Infused with natural coconut flavor, this cake has a moist tender crumb. It uses both coconut flour and toasted coconut, making it the perfect dessert for coconut lovers.

FOR THE CAKE

4 tablespoons (½ stick) unsalted butter, melted, plus more for greasing

½ cup unsweetened coconut flakes, for topping

1 cup coconut flour

½ cup granulated erythritol–monk fruit blend; *less sweet: ¼ cup*

2 teaspoons baking powder

¼ teaspoon sea salt

½ teaspoon vanilla extract

3 large eggs

1 cup full-fat sour cream

FOR THE GLAZE

¼ cup confectioners' erythritol–monk fruit blend

¼ teaspoon vanilla extract

2 to 3 tablespoons heavy (whipping) cream

TO MAKE THE CAKE

1. Preheat the oven to 325°F. Line the baking sheet with parchment paper. Grease the cake pan with butter and set aside.

2. Spread the unsweetened coconut flakes on the baking sheet in a thin, even layer and bake for 5 to 7 minutes, until golden brown. Remove from the oven and allow the flakes to cool on the baking sheet for 10 to 15 minutes. Increase the oven temperature to 350°F.

3. In the medium bowl, mix the coconut flour, granulated erythritol–monk fruit blend, baking powder, and salt. Stir in the melted butter, vanilla, and eggs, one at a time. Add the sour cream and mix until fully combined.

4. Pour the batter into the prepared cake pan and bake for 30 to 35 minutes, until lightly browned and a toothpick inserted into the center comes out clean.

5. While the cake bakes, in the small bowl, whisk together the confectioners' erythritol–monk fruit blend, vanilla, and 1 tablespoon of heavy cream. Add additional heavy cream, 1 tablespoon at a time, until the glaze is runny enough to drizzle easily.

6. Allow the cake to cool for at least 15 minutes before drizzling the glaze on top of the cake. Top with the toasted coconut. Cut into 12 slices and serve.

7. Store leftovers in an airtight container in the refrigerator for up to 5 days.

KEEP IN MIND: Instead of baking the coconut flakes, you can toast them in a dry large skillet over medium-low heat, stirring frequently for 3 to 5 minutes, until the flakes are golden brown.

Per serving: Calories: 157; **Total Fat:** 15g; **Total Carbohydrates:** 3g; **Net Carbs:** 1g; **Fiber:** 2g; **Protein:** 3g; Sweetener: 12g
Macros: **Fat:** 84%; **Protein:** 7%; **Carbs:** 9%

Carrot Cake

PREP TIME: 10 minutes COOK TIME: 40 minutes, plus 30 minutes to cool
EQUIPMENT: large mixing bowl, medium mixing bowl, electric mixer, 2 (9-inch) round cake pans,
parchment paper, cooling rack, toothpicks

A good carrot cake has a super moist crumb, is perfectly spiced, and topped with a rich cream cheese frosting. This cake delivers on all counts.

FOR THE CAKE

1 cup (2 sticks) unsalted butter, at room temperature, plus more for greasing
1 cup granulated erythritol–monk fruit blend; *less sweet: ¾ cup*
½ cup golden erythritol–monk fruit blend
5 large eggs, at room temperature
½ cup heavy (whipping) cream
2 cups loosely packed grated carrots
2½ cups finely milled almond flour, sifted
2½ teaspoons baking powder
2 tablespoons ground cinnamon
2 teaspoons ground ginger
½ teaspoon ground nutmeg
½ teaspoon sea salt
1½ cups coarsely chopped pecans, divided
½ cup unsweetened coconut flakes

FOR THE CREAM CHEESE FROSTING

12 ounces full-fat cream cheese, at room temperature
12 tablespoons (1½ sticks) unsalted butter, at room temperature
1¼ cups confectioners' erythritol–monk fruit blend
¾ cup heavy (whipping) cream

TO MAKE THE CAKE

1. Preheat the oven to 350°F. Grease the bottoms and sides of the cake pans with butter and line them with rounds of parchment paper.

2. In the large bowl, using an electric mixer on medium high, cream the butter, granulated erythritol–monk fruit blend, and golden erythritol–monk fruit blend for 2 to 3 minutes, until light and fluffy. Beat in the eggs, one at a time, mixing well after each addition, stopping and scraping the bowl once or twice, as needed. Add the heavy cream and combine well. Add the grated carrots and mix well until fully combined.

3. In a medium bowl, combine the almond flour, baking powder, cinnamon, ginger, nutmeg, and salt. Add the dry ingredients to the wet ingredients and combine well. Stir in 1 cup of pecans and the coconut. Divide the batter evenly between the two prepared cake pans.

4. Bake for 30 to 35 minutes, or until a toothpick inserted into the center of a cake comes out clean. Allow the cakes to cool in the pans for 10 minutes before transferring them to a cooling rack to cool thoroughly, about 20 minutes.

TO MAKE THE CREAM CHEESE FROSTING

5. While the cakes are baking, in a medium bowl, using an electric mixer on high, beat the cream cheese and butter until light and fluffy, 2 to 3 minutes, stopping and scraping the bowl once or twice, as needed. Add the confectioners' erythritol–monk fruit blend a little at a time, while mixing, then add the heavy cream a couple of tablespoons at a time, while mixing on high, until the frosting is light and fluffy, about 2 minutes.

6. Once the cakes have fully cooled, assemble the whole cake by adding one-third of the frosting on top of one of the cakes and place the second cake on top. Then use the remaining frosting to cover the top and sides. Top with the reserved ½ cup of pecans. Cut into 12 slices and serve.

7. Store leftovers in an airtight container in the refrigerator for up to 5 days or freeze for up to 3 weeks. If freezing, do not frost the cake; instead, store the frosting separately in an airtight container in the refrigerator for up to 5 days.

KEEP IN MIND: To get the best results when making the frosting, use the wire whipping attachment on your stand mixer or egg beaters on your handheld mixer.

Per serving: Calories: 683; Total Fat: 69g; Total Carbohydrates: 12g; Net Carbs: 7g; Fiber: 5g; Protein: 11g; Sweetener: 44g
Macros: Fat: 87%; Protein: 6%; Carbs: 7%

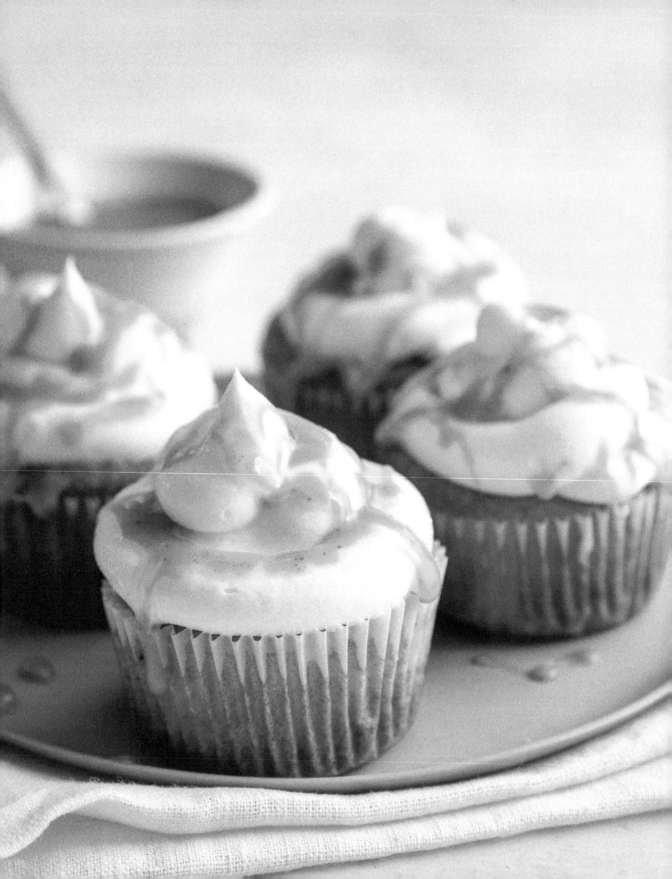

Salted Caramel Cupcakes

MAKES 12

PREP TIME: 20 minutes **COOK TIME:** 40 minutes, plus 20 minutes to cool
EQUIPMENT: medium mixing bowl, large mixing bowl, electric mixer, small saucepan, 12-cavity
muffin pan, toothpicks

These salty and sweet cupcakes make a scrumptious dessert for special occasions or any day of the week.

FOR THE CUPCAKES

1¼ cups finely milled almond flour, sifted

1 teaspoon baking powder

¼ teaspoon salt, plus more for topping

4 tablespoons (½ stick) unsalted butter, at room temperature

¾ cup granulated erythritol–monk fruit blend

3½ ounces full-fat cream cheese, at room temperature

1 teaspoon vanilla extract

4 large eggs, at room temperature

FOR THE CARAMEL SAUCE

2 tablespoons unsalted butter, at room temperature

1 cup allulose

¼ cup heavy (whipping) cream

FOR THE BUTTERCREAM

12 tablespoons (1½ sticks) unsalted butter, at room temperature

2 to 3 tablespoons heavy (whipping) cream

1 teaspoon vanilla extract

¼ teaspoon sea salt

1½ cups confectioners' erythritol–monk fruit blend

TO MAKE THE CUPCAKES

1. Preheat the oven to 350°F. Line the muffin pan with cupcake liners.

2. In the medium bowl, combine the almond flour, baking powder, and salt. Set aside.

3. In the large bowl, using an electric mixer on medium high, cream the butter with the granulated erythritol–monk fruit blend, stopping and scraping the bowl once or twice, as needed, until the mixture is light and fluffy and well incorporated.

4. Add the cream cheese and vanilla and mix well. Add the eggs, one at a time, making sure to mix well after each addition. Add the dry ingredients to the wet ingredients and mix well, until the batter is fully combined.

5. Fill the prepared muffin cups with the batter. Bake for 20 to 25 minutes, until golden brown and a toothpick inserted into a cupcake comes out clean. Cool on a cooling rack for 15 to 20 minutes or until completely cooled.

TO MAKE THE CARAMEL SAUCE

6. While the cupcakes bake, in the saucepan, brown the butter over medium heat, stirring constantly. Once the butter begins to foam and bubble, after 2 to 4 minutes, you should begin to see browned bits on the bottom of the pan. At this point, remove from the heat immediately and continue to stir until the butter turns to a golden amber color.

7. Add the allulose and return to the stove to cook over low heat. Once the sauce thickens, stir in the heavy cream, remove from the heat, and set aside.

TO MAKE THE BUTTERCREAM

8. In the large bowl, using an electric mixer on medium high, mix the butter, heavy cream, vanilla, and salt until well mixed, stopping and scraping the bowl once or twice, as needed. Add the confectioners' erythritol–monk fruit blend, 1 tablespoon at a time, beating well after each addition until fully incorporated.

9. Once the cupcakes have completely cooled, frost with the buttercream, drizzle on the caramel sauce, and top with salt to serve.

10. Store in an airtight container in the refrigerator for up to 5 days.

KEEP IN MIND: If your caramel separates try to coax it back together by removing it from the heat and cooling for about 10 minutes. Bring it back to the stove at a very low temperature and whisk in a tablespoon of water.

Per serving: **Calories:** 290: **Total Fat:** 29g: **Total Carbohydrates:** 3g: **Net Carbs:** 2g: **Fiber:** 1g: **Protein:** 5g
Sweetener: 51g
Macros: Fat: 90%: **Protein:** 7%: **Carbs:** 3%

Tiramisu

PREP TIME: 20 minutes COOK TIME: 45 minutes CHILL TIME: 8 hours
EQUIPMENT: large mixing bowl, medium mixing bowl, small mixing bowl, electric mixer, medium glass bowl, medium saucepan, 9-by-13-inch baking sheet, 9-by-5-inch loaf pan, sifter, parchment paper, pastry brush

Tiramisu without the guilt? Yes! This recipe doubles easily, which is great because your guests will be clamoring for seconds.

FOR THE CAKE

4 tablespoons (½ stick) unsalted butter, at room temperature
¾ cup granulated erythritol–monk fruit blend
4 ounces full-fat cream cheese, at room temperature
1 teaspoon vanilla extract
4 large eggs, at room temperature
1¼ cups finely milled almond flour, sifted
1 teaspoon baking powder
½ teaspoon sea salt

FOR THE CUSTARD

4 large egg yolks, at room temperature
½ cup granulated erythritol–monk fruit blend
¼ teaspoon sea salt
4 ounces mascarpone cheese
1 cup heavy (whipping) cream

FOR THE TOPPING

¼ cup espresso or strong coffee
2 tablespoons dark rum or ½ teaspoon rum extract
¼ cup unsweetened cocoa powder

TO MAKE THE CAKE

1. Preheat the oven to 350°F. Line the baking sheet with parchment paper and set aside.

2. In the large bowl, using an electric mixer on high, beat the butter and erythritol–monk fruit blend for 2 to 3 minutes, stopping and scraping the bowl once or twice, as needed, until light and fluffy and well incorporated. Add the cream cheese and vanilla and mix well. Add the eggs, one at a time, mixing well after each addition. Add the almond flour, baking powder, and salt and mix well until combined.

3. Spread the batter evenly into the prepared baking sheet. Bake for 25 to 30 minutes, until golden brown on top. Allow to cool fully, 15 to 20 minutes, before cutting into 1-by-3-inch slices to mimic ladyfingers.

TO MAKE THE CUSTARD

4. While the cake bakes, in the medium glass bowl, using an electric mixer on medium high, beat the egg yolks, erythritol–monk fruit blend, and salt, stopping and scraping the bowl once or twice, as needed, until thick and lemon colored.

5. Fill the saucepan with water and bring to a boil, then reduce the heat to a simmer. Put the glass bowl with the egg mixture over the simmering water, stirring constantly for 9 to 10 minutes, or until the mixture reaches a custard-like texture. Remove from the heat and stir in the mascarpone cheese.

6. In the medium bowl, using an electric mixer on high, beat the heavy cream for 3 to 5 minutes, stopping and scraping the bowl once or twice, as needed, until stiff peaks form. Gently fold the mascarpone mixture into the whipped cream. Set aside.

TO MAKE THE TOPPING

7. In the small bowl, combine the espresso and rum and set aside.

8. Using a sifter, sprinkle a layer of cocoa powder onto the bottom of the loaf pan. Place a layer of the cake "fingers" in the pan. Coat the layer with the coffee-rum mixture using a pastry brush. Follow by spreading one-quarter of the custard over the top. Repeat the layers of cake, coffee, and custard ending with the custard. Top with a generous coating of cocoa powder. Cover and refrigerate for at least 8 hours or overnight before serving.

9. Store leftovers in an airtight container in the refrigerator for up to 5 days.

INGREDIENT TIP: If you can't find mascarpone cheese, combine 8 ounces of cream cheese and ½ cup of sour cream for a substitute.

Per serving: Calories: 415; Total Fat: 39g; Total Carbohydrates: 7g; Net Carbs: 4g; Fiber: 3g; Protein: 11g; Sweetener: 30g
Macros: Fat: 84%; Protein: 10%; Carbs: 6%

No-Bake Chocolate Raspberry Cheesecake

SERVES 14

PREP TIME: 15 minutes COOK TIME: 10 minutes CHILL TIME: 4 hours
EQUIPMENT: large mixing bowl, electric mixer, 3 small microwave-safe bowls, 9-inch pie dish

If you are looking for an easy and elegant dessert, give this no-bake raspberry chocolate cheesecake a go. Just be prepared to make it again and again. You can swap the raspberries for your favorite keto-friendly fruit. For the sugar-free chocolate chips, I recommend Lily's Dark Chocolate Baking Chips.

FOR THE CRUST

4 tablespoons (½ stick) unsalted butter

2 ounces unsweetened baking chocolate

2 cups finely milled almond flour, sifted

¼ cup granulated erythritol–monk fruit blend; *less sweet: 3 tablespoons*

¼ teaspoon sea salt

FOR THE CHEESECAKE

4 tablespoons (½ stick) unsalted butter

2 ounces unsweetened baking chocolate, coarsely chopped

3 cups granulated erythritol–monk fruit blend; *less sweet: 2 cups*

20 ounces full-fat cream cheese, at room temperature

2 cups full-fat sour cream

¼ cup unsweetened cocoa powder

FOR THE TOPPING

1 tablespoon coconut oil

2 tablespoons sugar-free dark chocolate chips

1 cup chopped raspberries

TO MAKE THE CRUST

1. In a small microwave-safe bowl, melt the butter and baking chocolate together in the microwave in 30-second intervals. Add the almond flour, granulated erythritol–monk fruit blend, and salt to the melted chocolate and combine well. Press the mixture into the pie dish and put in the refrigerator to cool until ready to fill.

TO MAKE THE CHEESECAKE

2. In another small microwave-safe bowl, melt the butter and baking chocolate together in the microwave, in 30-second intervals, and set aside.

3. In the large bowl, using an electric mixer on medium high, beat the granulated erythritol–monk fruit blend, cream cheese, sour cream, and cocoa powder until well combined, stopping and scraping the bowl once or twice, as needed. Gradually fold in the chocolate and butter mixture until fully combined. Scrape the cheesecake batter into the chocolate crust and spread evenly.

TO MAKE THE TOPPING

4. In a third small microwave-safe bowl, melt the coconut oil and chocolate baking chips together in the microwave in 30-second intervals to make the chocolate sauce.

5. Top the cheesecake with the raspberries and drizzle with the chocolate sauce. Cover and refrigerate for at least 4 hours or overnight to set. Cut into 14 slices and serve.

6. Store leftovers in an airtight container in the refrigerator for up to 5 days.

KEEP IN MIND: For best results, I recommend making the pie the night before and allowing it to set overnight. I recommend using fresh raspberries, but if frozen is all that's available, allow them to thaw on the counter before adding them on top.

Per serving: Calories: 414; Total Fat: 40g; Total Carbohydrates: 10g; Net Carbs: 6g; Fiber: 4g; Protein: 8g; Sweetener: 44g
Macros: Fat: 84%; Protein: 7%; Carbs: 9%

Mini Cranberry Cheesecakes

SERVES 6

PREP TIME: 20 minutes COOK TIME: 1 hour 30 minutes, plus 2 hours 40 minutes to cool
CHILL TIME: 12 hours
EQUIPMENT: medium mixing bowl, large mixing bowl, electric mixer, 6 (4-inch) springform pans,
large roasting pan, medium saucepan, aluminum foil, plastic wrap, cooling rack

This velvety cheesecake with cranberry sauce will become a family favorite. If you prefer, you can make one large cheesecake in a 9-inch springform pan.

FOR THE CRUST

8 tablespoons (1 stick) unsalted butter,
  melted, plus more for greasing
2 cups finely milled almond flour
½ cup granulated erythritol–monk
  fruit blend
½ teaspoon sea salt

FOR THE CHEESECAKE

32 ounces full-fat cream cheese, at room
  temperature
1½ cups granulated erythritol–monk
  fruit blend
4 large eggs

16 ounces full-fat sour cream
1 teaspoon vanilla extract
¼ teaspoon sea salt
Unsalted butter, for greasing

FOR THE TOPPING

½ cup granulated erythritol–monk
  fruit blend
½ cup water
½ tablespoon freshly squeezed
  lemon juice
1 teaspoon freshly grated orange zest
½ teaspoon orange extract
6 ounces fresh or frozen cranberries

TO MAKE THE CRUST

1. Preheat the oven to 350°F. Lightly grease the bottom of the springform pans with butter.

2. In the medium bowl, mix the almond flour, erythritol–monk fruit blend, and salt and combine well. Add the melted butter and mix until fully incorporated.

3. Using the bottom of a glass cup, press the mixture evenly into the bottoms of the springform pans. Bake the crusts for 15 to 20 minutes, until lightly browned. Remove to a cooling rack for 15 to 20 minutes and reduce the oven temperature to 325°F.

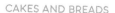

Mini Cranberry Cheesecakes CONTINUED

TO MAKE THE CHEESECAKE

4. In the large bowl, using an electric mixer on high, beat the cream cheese and erythritol–monk fruit blend until well incorporated. Reduce the speed of the mixer to medium low and add the eggs, one at a time, stopping and scraping the bowl once or twice, as needed. Add the sour cream, vanilla, and salt. Incorporation may take up to 5 minutes.

5. Use butter to lightly grease the sides of the cooled springform pans. Pour the cheesecake batter into the springforms and spread evenly. Wrap the bottoms and sides of the springform pans with heavy-duty aluminum foil. Put the wrapped pans in a large roasting pan large enough to accommodate the pans without touching the sides. Put the roasting pan with the cheesecakes in the oven and carefully pour in boiling water to halfway up the sides of the springform pans. Bake for 35 to 45 minutes, until the cheesecakes are set around the edges but the centers jiggle.

6. Cool the cheesecakes in the oven for 1 hour with the door slightly ajar. Then cool them on the cooling rack for at least 1 additional hour. Run a knife around the sides of the springform pans to release the cheesecakes.

7. Carefully wrap the cheesecakes with plastic wrap and allow them to chill in the refrigerator for at least 12 hours and up to 36 hours before serving.

TO MAKE THE TOPPING

8. In the saucepan, bring the erythritol–monk fruit blend, water, lemon juice, orange zest, and orange extract to a boil. Add the cranberries and allow the mixture to simmer for 10 to 15 minutes, stirring occasionally. The sauce is ready when the cranberries pop and the sauce thickens. Allow the sauce to cool for 15 to 20 minutes.

9. Spread the topping evenly on each mini cheesecake and serve.

10. Store leftovers in an airtight container in the refrigerator for up to 5 days.

Per serving: Calories: 1045; Total Fat: 101g; Total Carbohydrates: 19g; Net Carbs: 13g; Fiber: 6g; Protein: 22g; Sweetener: 80g
Macros: Fat: 85%; Protein: 8%; Carbs: 7%

Classic Cheesecake

PREP TIME: 15 minutes **COOK TIME:** 1 hour 30 minutes, plus 2 hours 30 minutes to cool
CHILL TIME: 12 hours
EQUIPMENT: medium mixing bowl, large mixing bowl, small mixing bowl, electric mixer, 9-inch
springform pan, large roasting pan, aluminum foil, plastic wrap, cooling rack

This creamy cheesecake topped with a traditional sour-cream topping makes a great base for any number of garnishes. Make a classic strawberry topping (see tip) or try a peanut butter and chocolate drizzle.

FOR THE CRUST

8 tablespoons (1 stick) unsalted butter, melted, plus more for greasing
2 cups finely milled almond flour
½ cup granulated erythritol–monk fruit blend
½ teaspoon sea salt

FOR THE CHEESECAKE

32 ounces full-fat cream cheese, at room temperature
1½ cups granulated erythritol–monk fruit blend

4 large eggs
16 ounces full-fat sour cream
1 teaspoon vanilla extract
¼ teaspoon sea salt
Unsalted butter, for greasing

FOR THE SOUR CREAM TOPPING

1½ cups sour cream
3 tablespoons granulated erythritol–monk fruit blend
½ teaspoon vanilla extract

TO MAKE THE CRUST

1. Preheat the oven to 350°F. Lightly grease the bottom of the springform pan with butter.

2. In the medium bowl, mix the almond flour, erythritol–monk fruit blend, and salt and combine well. Add the melted butter and mix until fully incorporated. Once combined, add the mixture to the bottom of the springform pan. Use the bottom of a glass cup to press the mixture evenly into the pan.

3. Bake the crust for 20 to 25 minutes, until lightly browned. Move the crust to the cooling rack and allow the crust to cool for 15 to 20 minutes. Leave the oven on and reduce the oven temperature to 325°F.

TO MAKE THE CHEESECAKE

4. In the large bowl, using an electric mixer on high, beat the cream cheese and erythritol–monk fruit blend until well incorporated. Reduce the speed to medium low and add the eggs, one at a time, stopping and scraping the bowl once or twice, as needed. Add the sour cream, vanilla, and salt. Combine the mixture until fully incorporated and velvety smooth. This may take up to 5 minutes. Stop and scrape the bowl a couple of times during this process as well.

5. Use butter to lightly grease the sides of the cooled springform pan with the crust. Pour the cheesecake batter into the almond crust and spread evenly. Wrap the bottom and sides of the springform pan with heavy-duty aluminum foil. Put the wrapped springform pan in a roasting pan large enough to accommodate the springform pan without touching the sides.

6. Put the roasting pan in the oven and carefully pour in boiling water to halfway up the sides of the springform pan. Bake for 1 hour to 1 hour 10 minutes, until the cheesecake is set around the edges but the center jiggles.

7. Allow the cheesecake to cool in the oven for 1 hour with the oven off and door slightly ajar.

8. Move the cheesecake to the cooling rack to further cool on the kitchen counter for at least 1 additional hour. Once fully cooled, run a knife around the sides of the springform pan to release the cheesecake.

9. Carefully wrap the cheesecake with plastic wrap and chill in the refrigerator for at least 12 hours and up to 36 hours before serving.

TO MAKE THE SOUR CREAM TOPPING

10. In the small bowl, combine the sour cream, erythritol–monk fruit blend, and vanilla. Spread evenly on top of the cheesecake right before serving, cut into 14 slices, and serve.

11. Store leftovers in an airtight container in the refrigerator for up to 5 days.

VARIATION TIP: Instead of a sour cream topping, make a quick and easy strawberry topping by combining 2 cups of sliced fresh strawberries with 2 tablespoons of granulated erythritol–monk fruit blend. This will naturally create a sauce as it sits.

Per serving: **Calories:** 413: **Total Fat:** 41g: **Total Carbohydrates:** 4g: **Net Carbs:** 4g: **Fiber:** 0g: **Protein:** 7g: **Sweetener:** 30g
Macros: Fat: 89%: **Protein:** 7%: **Carbs:** 4%

Nut-Free Pumpkin Bread

PREP TIME: 15 minutes COOK TIME: 55 minutes, plus 30 minutes to cool
EQUIPMENT: large mixing bowl, electric mixer, 9-by-5-inch loaf pan, cooling rack, toothpicks

This pumpkin bread is easy to make and perfectly spiced. Enjoy it plain or with a pat of butter. If you can have nuts, add ¼ cup of finely chopped walnuts to the mix in the final step.

4 tablespoons (½ stick) unsalted butter, melted, plus more for greasing

1 cup granulated erythritol–monk fruit blend; *less sweet:* ½ cup

¾ cup canned pumpkin puree

1 teaspoon vanilla extract

4 large eggs, at room temperature

1½ cups sunflower seed flour

½ cup golden flaxseed meal, reground in a clean coffee grinder

1½ teaspoons baking powder

1 tablespoon psyllium husk powder

2 teaspoons ground cinnamon

1½ teaspoons ground ginger

½ teaspoon ground nutmeg

¼ teaspoon ground cloves

¼ teaspoon sea salt

1. Preheat the oven to 350°F. Grease the loaf pan with butter and set aside.

2. In the large bowl, using an electric mixer on medium high, beat the butter, erythritol–monk fruit blend, pumpkin puree, and vanilla until well blended, stopping and scraping the bowl once or twice, as needed. Add the eggs, one at time, stopping and scraping the bowl once or twice, as needed. Add the sunflower seed flour, flaxseed meal, baking powder, psyllium husk powder, cinnamon, ginger, nutmeg, cloves, and salt.

3. Spread the batter into the prepared loaf pan. Bake for 40 to 55 minutes, or until a toothpick inserted into the center comes out clean. Let cool for 10 minutes in the pan.

4. Remove the pumpkin bread from the pan and allow to cool 15 to 20 minutes.

5. Store leftovers in an airtight container in the refrigerator for up to 5 days or freeze for 3 weeks.

Per serving: Calories: 195; Total Fat: 17g; Total Carbohydrates: 7g; Net Carbs: 3g; Fiber: 4g; Protein: 6g; Sweetener: 12g
Macros: Fat: 75%; Protein: 12%; Carbs: 13%

Chocolate Chip Scones

MAKES 10

PREP TIME: 10 minutes **COOK TIME:** 30 minutes
EQUIPMENT: large mixing bowl, electric mixer, 9-inch cast-iron skillet, toothpicks

Chocolate chips steal the show in these melt-in-your-mouth scones. These are perfect for an on-the-go breakfast or leisurely brunch.

4 tablespoons (½ stick) unsalted butter, melted, plus more for greasing

½ cup granulated erythritol–monk fruit blend

3 large eggs

½ cup full-fat sour cream

1½ cups finely milled almond flour, sifted

½ cup coconut flour

1½ teaspoons baking powder

¼ teaspoon sea salt

4 ounces sugar-free chocolate chips

2 tablespoons confectioners' erythritol–monk fruit blend, for dusting (optional)

1. Preheat the oven to 375°F. Grease the cast-iron skillet with butter and set aside.

2. In the large bowl, using an electric mixer on medium high, mix the granulated erythritol–monk fruit blend, melted butter, and eggs until well combined, stopping and scraping the bowl once or twice, as needed. Add the sour cream and mix well. Add the almond flour, coconut flour, baking powder, and salt, then stir until fully combined. Fold the sugar-free chocolate chips into the batter.

3. Spread the batter evenly into the cast-iron skillet. Bake for 25 to 30 minutes, or until a toothpick inserted into the center comes out clean. Allow the scones to cool completely. Dust with confectioners' erythritol–monk fruit blend (if using) and cut into 10 wedges before serving.

4. Store leftovers in an airtight container in the refrigerator for up to 5 days or freeze for up to 3 weeks.

VARIATION TIP: Change up the flavor by adding your favorite extracts: 1 teaspoon of orange extract would make for a great orange-chocolate scone.

Per serving (1 scone): Calories: 268; Total Fat: 24g; Total Carbohydrates: 8g; Net Carbs: 4g; Fiber: 4g; Protein: 7g; Sweetener: 10g
Macros: Fat: 78%; Protein: 10%; Carbs: 12%

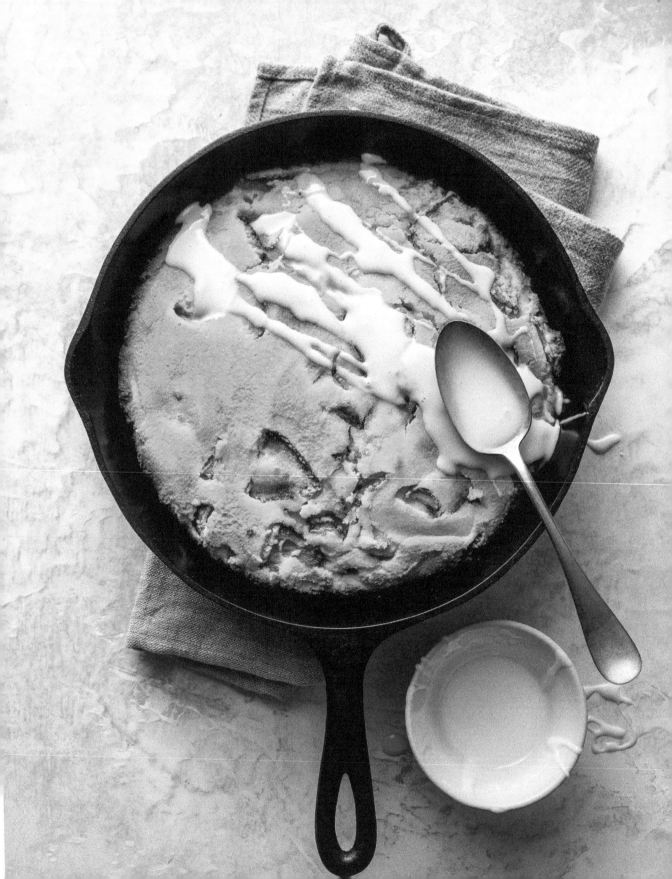

Strawberry Rhubarb Scones

MAKES 10

PREP TIME: 10 minutes **COOK TIME:** 30 minutes, plus 20 minutes to cool
EQUIPMENT: large mixing bowl, small mixing bowl, electric mixer, 9-inch cast-iron skillet, toothpicks

Tangy rhubarb and sweet strawberries make these scones special. If you don't have a super-sweet tooth like me, you can omit the icing, but I find it balances out the tartness of the rhubarb.

FOR THE SCONES

4 tablespoons (½ stick) unsalted butter, melted, plus more for greasing
½ cup granulated erythritol–monk fruit blend
3 large eggs
½ cup full-fat sour cream
1½ cups finely milled almond flour, sifted
½ cup coconut flour
1½ teaspoons baking powder
¼ teaspoon sea salt

¾ cup fresh or frozen strawberries, thinly sliced
¾ cup fresh or frozen rhubarb, thinly sliced

FOR THE ICING

½ cup confectioners' erythritol–monk fruit blend
½ teaspoon vanilla extract
3 to 4 tablespoons heavy (whipping) cream

TO MAKE THE SCONES

1. Preheat the oven to 375°F. Grease the cast-iron skillet with butter and set aside.

2. In the large bowl, using an electric mixer on medium high, blend the granulated erythritol–monk fruit blend, melted butter, and eggs, stopping and scraping the bowl once or twice, as needed. Add the sour cream and mix well. Add the almond flour, coconut flour, baking powder, and salt, then stir until fully combined. Fold the strawberries and rhubarb into the batter.

3. Spread the batter evenly into the cast-iron skillet. Bake for 25 to 30 minutes, or until an inserted toothpick comes out clean. Cool completely, about 20 minutes.

TO MAKE THE ICING

4. In a small bowl, combine the confectioners' erythritol–monk fruit blend and vanilla. Add the heavy cream, starting with 1 tablespoon. Drizzle the icing onto the cooled scones and cut into 10 wedges before serving.

5. Store leftovers in an airtight container in the refrigerator for up to 5 days or freeze without the icing for up to 3 weeks.

Per serving (1 scone): **Calories:** 222; **Total Fat:** 20g; **Total Carbohydrates:** 6g; **Net Carbs:** 3g; **Fiber:** 3g; **Protein:** 6g; **Sweetener:** 19g
Macros: Fat: 79%; **Protein:** 10%; **Carbs:** 11%

Blueberry Muffins

PREP TIME: 5 minutes **COOK TIME:** 25 minutes, plus 20 minutes to cool
EQUIPMENT: large mixing bowl, small mixing bowl, electric mixer, 12-cavity muffin pan, toothpicks

These blueberry muffins are perfect for weekend brunches or afternoon snacks. A lemon icing takes them over the top. Friends and family won't say no to one of these muffins!

FOR THE MUFFINS
Unsalted butter, for greasing
4 ounces full-fat cream cheese, at room
  temperature
¼ cup coconut oil, solid
1 cup plus 2 tablespoons granulated
  erythritol–monk fruit blend; *less*
  sweet: ¾ cup
4 large eggs, at room temperature
1¼ cups finely milled almond flour, sifted
1 teaspoon baking powder

½ teaspoon vanilla extract
¼ teaspoon sea salt
1 cup fresh or frozen blueberries

FOR THE ICING
¼ cup confectioners' erythritol–monk
  fruit blend
¼ teaspoon lemon extract
2 to 3 tablespoons heavy
  (whipping) cream

TO MAKE THE MUFFINS

1. Preheat the oven to 350°F. Grease the muffin pan generously with butter and set aside.

2. In the large bowl, using an electric mixer on high, beat the cream cheese and coconut oil for 1 to 2 minutes, stopping and scraping the bowl once or twice, as needed, until light and fluffy. Add the granulated erythritol–monk fruit blend and continue to mix well. Add the eggs, one at a time, mixing well after each addition.

3. Stir in the almond flour, baking powder, vanilla, and salt and mix well. Fold in the blueberries and mix until the batter is fully incorporated.

4. Pour the batter evenly into the prepared muffin cups and bake for 20 to 25 minutes, or until a toothpick inserted into the center of a muffin comes out clean. Allow to cool for 15 to 20 minutes.

TO MAKE THE ICING

5. In a small bowl, combine the confectioners' erythritol–monk fruit blend and lemon extract. Add the heavy cream, starting with 1 tablespoon. Add additional cream if the icing is too thick. Once the muffins have fully cooled, drizzle with icing.

6. Store leftovers in an airtight container in the refrigerator for up to 5 days or freeze without the glaze for up to 3 weeks.

VARIATION TIP: If you're wanting a less sweet muffin, but don't want to lose the lemony flavor, omit the icing, but grate the zest of 1 lemon and stir the zest into the muffin batter before baking.

Per serving: **Calories:** 177; **Total Fat:** 16g; **Total Carbohydrates:** 5g; **Net Carbs:** 3g; **Fiber:** 2g; **Protein:** 5g; **Sweetener:** 20g
Macros: Fat: 79%; **Protein:** 11%; **Carbs:** 10%

Dairy-Free Cranberry Muffins

MAKES 12

PREP TIME: 10 minutes **COOK TIME:** 25 minutes, plus 20 minutes to cool
EQUIPMENT: 2 large mixing bowls, electric mixer, 12-cavity muffin pan, toothpicks

These dairy-free muffins are moist, flavorful, and healthy. Fresh or frozen cranberries work equally well. If you're opting for frozen, you don't need to thaw the berries before adding them to the batter.

½ cup coconut oil, solid, plus more for greasing

¾ cup granulated erythritol–monk fruit blend

2 large eggs, at room temperature

¼ cup coconut or almond milk

½ teaspoon orange extract

1½ cups finely milled almond flour, sifted

1¼ teaspoons baking powder

1 teaspoon ground cinnamon

¼ teaspoon ground nutmeg

¼ teaspoon sea salt

1 cup fresh or frozen cranberries

1. Preheat the oven 350°F. Grease the muffin pan generously with coconut oil and set aside.

2. In a large bowl, using an electric mixer on medium high, cream the coconut oil and erythritol–monk fruit blend for 1 to 2 minutes, stopping and scraping the bowl once or twice, as needed, until light and fluffy. Beat in the eggs, one at a time. Add the coconut milk and orange extract and combine well.

3. In another large bowl, combine the almond flour, baking powder, cinnamon, nutmeg, and salt. Add the dry ingredients to the wet ingredients and mix well. Fold in the cranberries.

4. Pour the batter evenly into the muffin cups. Bake for 20 to 25 minutes, or until a toothpick inserted in a muffin comes out clean. Allow to cool for 15 to 20 minutes before serving.

5. Store in an airtight container in the refrigerator for up to 5 days or freeze for up to 3 weeks.

VARIATION TIP: For a tasty, nutty cinnamon muffin, swap pecans for the cranberries.

Per serving: Calories: 173; Total Fat: 17g; Total Carbohydrates: 4g; Net Carbs: 2g; Fiber: 2g; Protein: 4g; Sweetener: 12g
Macros: Fat: 83%; Protein: 8%; Carbs: 9%

Dairy-Free Chocolate Donuts

MAKES 12

PREP TIME: 10 minutes **COOK TIME:** 30 minutes, plus 20 minutes to cool
EQUIPMENT: large mixing bowl, electric mixer, small microwave-safe bowl, 12-by-17-inch baking sheet, 2 (6-cavity) silicone donut molds, parchment paper, toothpicks

These donuts are perfect for gatherings and parties because they are not only keto-friendly but also dairy-free! Most important, they are rich and chocolatey. If you'd rather not go chocolate all the way, swap out the icing for my Dairy-Free Vanilla Icing on page 166.

FOR THE DONUTS

¼ cup coconut oil, melted, plus more for greasing

2 cups granulated erythritol–monk fruit blend

2 cups finely milled almond flour, sifted

¾ cup coconut flour

¾ cup unsweetened cocoa powder

1½ teaspoons baking powder

1½ teaspoons baking soda

½ teaspoon sea salt

1 cup full-fat coconut milk or almond milk

1 cup boiling water

1 teaspoon vanilla extract

3 large eggs

FOR THE ICING

4 ounces unsweetened baking chocolate, coarsely chopped

½ cup confectioners' erythritol–monk fruit blend

2 tablespoons coconut oil

¼ teaspoon sea salt

TO MAKE THE DONUTS

1. Preheat the oven to 350°F. Grease the silicone molds well with coconut oil.

2. In the large bowl, combine the granulated erythritol–monk fruit blend, almond flour, coconut flour, cocoa powder, baking powder, baking soda, and salt. Add the coconut milk, boiling water, coconut oil, and vanilla. Add the eggs, one at a time, mixing well after each addition. Using an electric mixer on medium, mix the batter until fully incorporated, stopping and scraping the bowl once or twice, as needed.

3. Pour the batter into the prepared molds and bake for 25 to 30 minutes, until a toothpick inserted in a donut comes out clean. Allow to fully cool, 15 to 20 minutes, before taking the donuts out of the molds.

4. Line the baking sheet with parchment paper and set aside.

5. In the small microwave-safe bowl, melt the baking chocolate in the microwave in 30-second intervals. Add the confectioners' erythritol–monk fruit blend, coconut oil, and salt and combine until silky smooth.

6. Once the donuts are fully cooled, dip each of them into the chocolate icing, taking care to evenly coat the tops. Place them on the prepared baking sheet and allow them to chill in the refrigerator until ready to serve.

7. Store leftovers in an airtight container in the refrigerator for up to 5 days.

KEEP IN MIND: To make adding the batter to molds easier and cleaner, put the batter in a large resealable bag and cut the tip to make a pastry bag for piping the batter.

Per serving: **Calories:** 309; **Total Fat:** 28g; **Total Carbohydrates:** 11g; **Net Carbs:** 5g; **Fiber:** 6g; **Protein:** 8g; **Sweetener:** 40g
Macros: Fat: 79%; **Protein:** 9%; **Carbs:** 12%

Poppy Seed Pound Cake

SERVES 12

PREP TIME: 10 minutes **COOK TIME:** 40 minutes
EQUIPMENT: medium mixing bowl, large mixing bowl, electric mixer, 9-by-5-inch loaf pan, parchment paper, toothpicks

This poppy seed pound cake has a lemony flavor and delightful crunch. It's an excellent option for breakfast or a coffee or tea break.

4 tablespoons (½ stick) unsalted butter, at room temperature, plus more for greasing

1¼ cups finely milled almond flour, sifted

1 teaspoon baking powder

¼ teaspoon salt

¾ cup granulated erythritol–monk fruit blend; *less sweet: ½ cup*

3½ ounces full-fat cream cheese, at room temperature

1 teaspoon lemon extract

4 large eggs, at room temperature

1½ tablespoons poppy seeds

1. Preheat the oven to 350°F. Grease the loaf pan with butter, line with parchment paper, and set aside.

2. In the medium bowl, combine the almond flour, baking powder, and salt. Set aside.

3. In the large bowl, using an electric mixer on medium high, cream the butter and erythritol–monk fruit blend for 1 to 2 minutes, until light and fluffy.

4. Add the cream cheese and lemon extract and mix well. Add the eggs, one at a time, making sure to mix well after each addition. Add the dry ingredients to the wet ingredients and mix well. Stir in the poppy seeds and mix well.

5. Pour the batter into the prepared loaf pan. Bake for 30 to 40 minutes, until golden brown and a toothpick inserted into the center comes out clean. Let cool for 10 to 15 minutes, then cut into 12 slices and serve.

6. Store leftovers in an airtight container in the refrigerator for up to 5 days or freeze for up to 3 weeks.

VARIATION TIP: For an on-the-go, portion-controlled treat, line 12 cups of a muffin pan, fill with batter, and bake for 20 to 25 minutes.

Per serving: Calories: 149; Total Fat: 14g; Total Carbohydrates: 3g; Net Carbs: 1g; Fiber: 2g; Protein: 5g; Sweetener: 12g
Macros: Fat: 79%; Protein: 13%; Carbs: 8%

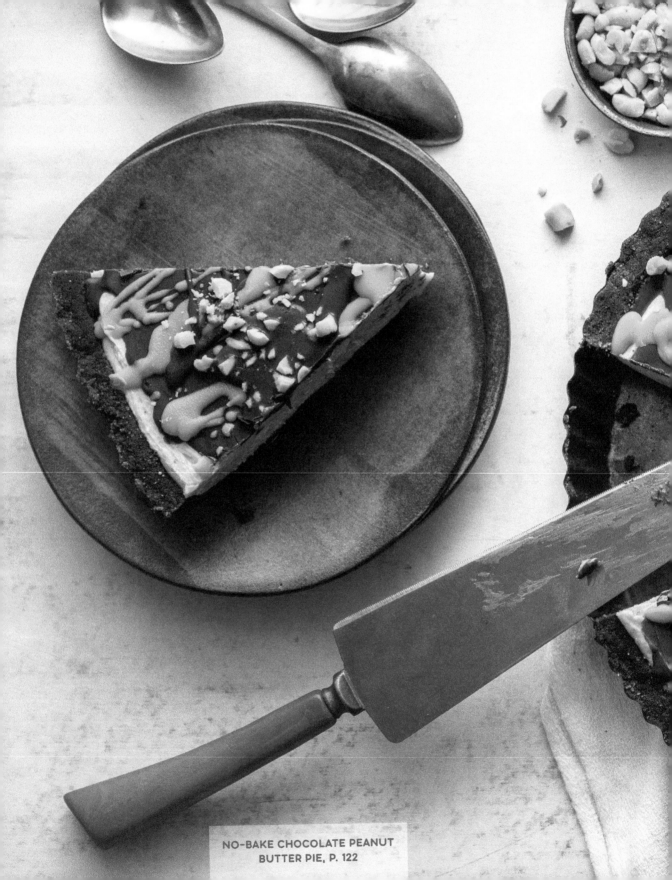

NO-BAKE CHOCOLATE PEANUT
BUTTER PIE, P. 122

Pies and Tarts

No-Bake Chocolate Peanut Butter Pie 122

Pumpkin Pie 124

Fudge Pie 126

"Apple" Pie 128

Coconut Cream Pie 130

Raspberry Mousse Tart 132

Lemon Curd Tartlets 134

Cinnamon Pecan "Apple" Crisp 136

Mixed Berry Crisp 139

Blueberry Crumble 140

Strawberry Rhubarb Cobbler 141

No-Bake Chocolate Peanut Butter Pie

SERVES 10

PREP TIME: 10 minutes **COOK TIME:** 5 minutes, plus 20 minutes to cool
CHILL TIME: 2 hours 45 minutes
EQUIPMENT: medium mixing bowl, large mixing bowl, electric mixer, 2 small microwave-safe bowls,
9-inch pie dish

This dreamy no-bake pie features a chocolate cookie crust and peanut butter filling. A chocolate–peanut butter ganache topping makes it your low-carb answer to any sweet craving. Feel free to swap the peanut butter for your favorite nut or seed butter.

FOR THE CRUST

8 tablespoons (1 stick) unsalted butter,
  melted, plus more for greasing
2 cups finely milled almond flour, sifted
½ cup confectioners' erythritol–monk
  fruit blend
½ cup unsweetened cocoa powder
½ teaspoon salt

FOR THE FILLING

12 ounces full-fat cream cheese, at room
  temperature
1 cup all-natural peanut butter (no
  added sugar or salt)
½ cup confectioners' erythritol–monk
  fruit blend; *less sweet: ¼ cup*

2 teaspoons vanilla extract
¼ teaspoon sea salt
1 cup heavy (whipping) cream

FOR THE CHOCOLATE TOPPING

⅓ cup sugar-free chocolate baking chips
1 tablespoon coconut oil, melted

FOR THE PEANUT BUTTER DRIZZLE

2 tablespoons all-natural creamy peanut
  butter (no added sugar or salt)
1 tablespoon coconut oil, melted
¼ cup crushed salted peanuts,
  for garnish

TO MAKE THE CRUST

1. Lightly grease the pie dish with butter.

2. In the medium bowl, combine the almond flour, confectioners' erythritol–monk fruit blend, cocoa powder, and salt. Stir in the melted butter and mix well. Press the mixture into the bottom of the prepared pie dish and up the sides.

3. Freeze to set for 15 to 20 minutes.

TO MAKE THE FILLING

4. In the large bowl, using an electric mixer on high, beat the cream cheese, peanut butter, confectioners' erythritol–monk fruit blend, vanilla, and salt, stopping and scraping the bowl once or twice, as needed. Add the heavy cream and combine until well incorporated.

5. Spread the pie filling evenly over the crust and put back in the freezer for 15 to 20 minutes.

TO MAKE THE CHOCOLATE TOPPING

6. In a small microwave-safe bowl, melt the chocolate baking chips and coconut oil in the microwave in 30-second intervals.

7. Allow the mixture to cool slightly, 5 to 10 minutes, before gently spreading across the surface of the frozen pie. Reserve a couple of tablespoons of the chocolate mixture to drizzle later.

TO MAKE THE PEANUT BUTTER DRIZZLE

8. In another small microwave-safe bowl, melt the peanut butter and coconut oil in the microwave in 30-second intervals. Allow the mixture to cool slightly, 5 to 10 minutes, before drizzling across the surface of the pie.

9. Drizzle the remaining chocolate topping across the pie and garnish with the crushed peanuts.

10. Put the pie in the freezer for 30 minutes or in the refrigerator for 2 hours to set.

11. Store leftovers in the refrigerator for up to 5 days or in the freezer for up to 2 weeks.

Per serving: Calories: 664; Total Fat: 60g; Total Carbohydrates: 15g; Net Carbs: 8g; Fiber: 7g; Protein: 16g Sweetener: 19g
Macros: Fat: 82%; Protein: 10%; Carbs: 8%

Pumpkin Pie

PREP TIME: 10 minutes **COOK TIME:** 1 hour 5 minutes, plus 40 minutes to cool
EQUIPMENT: medium mixing bowl, large mixing bowl, electric mixer, 9-inch pie dish,
cooling rack, toothpicks

During the holidays, temptations reach an all-time high. Thankfully, this keto pumpkin pie will make it easy to resist traditional desserts. If you worry about your crust browning too quickly in the oven, add aluminum foil to the edges midway through baking. Serve this pie at your next Thanksgiving with my Whipped Cream on page 167, and everyone will thank you.

FOR THE CRUST

1 cup (2 sticks) unsalted butter, melted
  and cooled, plus more for greasing

1½ cups coconut flour

4 large eggs

½ teaspoon sea salt

FOR THE FILLING

1 (15-ounce) can pumpkin puree

¾ cup heavy (whipping) cream

¾ cup granulated erythritol–monk
  fruit blend

3 large eggs

1 teaspoon vanilla extract

1 teaspoon ground cinnamon

½ teaspoon ground ginger

¼ teaspoon ground nutmeg

¼ teaspoon ground allspice

¼ teaspoon sea salt

TO MAKE THE CRUST

1. Preheat the oven to 350°F. Lightly grease the pie dish with butter.

2. In the medium bowl, mix the coconut flour, melted butter, eggs, and salt, until the dough forms. Press the dough into the bottom and sides of the prepared pie dish.

3. Bake for 25 minutes, or until lightly browned. Set the pie dish on the cooling rack for 15 to 20 minutes. Increase the oven temperature to 425°F.

4. In the large bowl, using an electric mixer on medium, mix the pumpkin puree, heavy cream, erythritol–monk fruit blend, eggs, vanilla, cinnamon, ginger, nutmeg, allspice, and salt until fully combined, stopping and scraping the bowl once or twice, as needed.

5. Pour the pie filling into the crust and bake for 15 minutes, then reduce the oven temperature to 350°F and bake the pie for 30 to 35 minutes, until a toothpick inserted into the center comes out clean. Put the pie on the cooling rack for 15 to 20 minutes before cutting it into 10 slices and serving.

6. Store leftovers in an airtight container in the refrigerator for up to 5 days.

SPICE IT UP: For an extra festive pie, top with Pralines (page 27) once baked. This takes your pie from holiday classic to unforgettable.

Per serving: **Calories:** 364; **Total Fat:** 32g; **Total Carbohydrates:** 11g; **Net Carbs:** 5g; **Fiber:** 6g; **Protein:** 8g
Sweetener: 14g
Macros: Fat: 80%; **Protein:** 8%; **Carbs:** 12%

Fudge Pie

PREP TIME: 15 minutes **COOK TIME:** 50 minutes, plus 20 minutes to cool
EQUIPMENT: large mixing bowl, medium mixing bowl, small microwave-safe bowl, electric mixer, 9-inch pie dish, toothpicks

The finest fudge pie—sans the sugar crash—is yours with this easy-to-make recipe. Chocolate lovers, you're in for a real treat. For an extra chocolicious kick, serve this pie with my Dairy-Free Mocha Ice "Cream" on page 152.

FOR THE CRUST

1 cup (2 sticks) unsalted butter, melted and cooled, plus more for greasing

1½ cups coconut flour

4 large eggs, at room temperature

2 teaspoons granulated erythritol–monk fruit blend

½ teaspoon sea salt

FOR THE FILLING

4 ounces unsweetened baking chocolate, coarsely chopped

8 tablespoons (1 stick) unsalted butter, at room temperature

3 large eggs, at room temperature

1 cup granulated erythritol–monk fruit blend

¼ teaspoon sea salt

TO MAKE THE CRUST

1. Preheat the oven to 360°F. Grease the pie dish with butter.

2. In the large bowl, combine the coconut flour, melted butter, eggs, erythritol–monk fruit blend, and salt. Mix just until the dough forms.

3. Pat and press the dough into the bottom and sides of the prepared pie dish and bake for 15 minutes. The piecrust will not be fully cooked at this point because it will go back into the oven once the fudge filling is added.

4. While the crust bakes, in the small microwave-safe bowl, melt the baking chocolate and butter together in the microwave in 30-second intervals. Allow the chocolate mixture to cool completely, about 20 minutes.

5. In the medium bowl, using an electric mixer on high, beat the eggs, erythritol–monk fruit blend, and salt for about 3 minutes, until the mixture is thick and pale yellow. Reduce the speed to medium low and add the cooled chocolate to the egg mixture, blending fully.

6. Pour the fudge filling into the piecrust and bake for 30 minutes, until the fudge filling is set and a toothpick inserted into the center comes out with moist crumbs. Cut into 10 slices and serve warm or cold.

7. Store leftovers in an airtight container in the refrigerator for up to 5 days.

KEEP IN MIND: Wetting your hands will make it easier to pat the crust in place. When baking the piecrust, cover the edges of the pie with foil to prevent it from browning too much.

Per serving: **Calories:** 438; **Total Fat:** 44g; **Total Carbohydrates:** 6g; **Net Carbs:** 2g; **Fiber:** 4g; **Protein:** 7g; **Sweetener:** 19g
Macros: Fat: 87%; **Protein:** 7%; **Carbs:** 6%

"Apple" Pie

PREP TIME: 20 minutes **COOK TIME:** 1 hour 10 minutes, plus 20 minutes to cool
EQUIPMENT: medium mixing bowl, large mixing bowl, medium saucepan, 9-inch pie dish, parchment paper, rolling pin

This mock apple pie delivers all of the flavors of apple pie without any sugar or gluten. If you can't find chayote squash, see the tip in the Cinnamon Pecan "Apple" Crisp (page 136) for using zucchini instead.

FOR THE FILLING

5 chayote squash

¾ cup granulated erythritol–monk fruit blend; *less sweet:* ½ cup

2 tablespoons freshly squeezed lemon juice

2 tablespoons ground cinnamon

½ teaspoon ground ginger

¼ teaspoon ground nutmeg

1½ teaspoons cream of tartar

FOR THE CRUST

2 cups (4 sticks) unsalted butter, melted and cooled, plus 2 tablespoons, chilled and sliced, plus more for greasing

3 cups coconut flour

4 teaspoons granulated erythritol–monk fruit blend

1 teaspoon sea salt

3 cups coconut flour

8 large eggs, at room temperature

TO MAKE THE FILLING

1. In the saucepan, cover the chayote squash with water and boil for 25 to 30 minutes. They should be firm but cooked through. Allow the squash to cool, 15 to 20 minutes, before peeling and cutting into ¼-inch-thick slices.

2. In the medium bowl, combine the squash, erythritol–monk fruit blend, lemon juice, cinnamon, ginger, nutmeg, and cream of tartar, mix until well incorporated, and set aside.

3. Preheat the oven to 375°F. Grease the pie dish with butter and set aside.

4. In the large bowl, combine the coconut flour, erythritol–monk fruit blend, and salt. Add the cooled melted butter and eggs and mix just until the dough forms.

5. Divide the dough in half to make the top and bottom crusts. Roll out half of the dough between two sheets of parchment paper with a rolling pin. Transfer the crust to the pie dish. Be careful to smooth out any cracks by pressing the dough together. Roll out the second half and set aside.

6. Add the filling to the pie dish, spread evenly, and dot with the sliced butter. Very carefully, add the second crust on top. Press the edges together with a fork to seal the two crusts together and cut several small slits in the middle to allow the pie to vent while baking.

7. Bake for 35 to 40 minutes, until the crust is slightly golden. Cut into 10 slices and serve warm or cold.

8. Store leftovers in an airtight container in the refrigerator for up to 5 days.

KEEP IN MIND: The dough for the crust tends to be very fragile and should be handled very delicately. Patience is key when moving the rolled-out dough. If any breaks occur, press them back together with your hands.

Per serving: Calories: 518; Total Fat: 50g; Total Carbohydrates: 9g; Net Carbs: 5g; Fiber: 4g; Protein: 8g Sweetener: 15g
Macros: Fat: 87%; Protein: 6%; Carbs: 7%

Coconut Cream Pie

PREP TIME: 15 minutes **COOK TIME:** 45 minutes, plus 30 minutes to cool **CHILL TIME:** 4 hours
EQUIPMENT: 2 large mixing bowls, electric mixer, medium skillet, medium saucepan, 9-inch pie dish

This pie has a luscious coconut custard nestled in a coconut-flour crust. Billows of whipped cream and a sprinkling of toasted coconut top this creamy confection that's a dream to eat on a summer day.

FOR THE CRUST

1 cup (2 sticks) unsalted butter, melted
  and cooled, plus more for greasing
1½ cups coconut flour
4 large eggs, at room temperature
2 teaspoons granulated erythritol–monk
  fruit blend
½ teaspoon sea salt

FOR THE FILLING

⅓ cup heavy (whipping) cream, whisked
  until stiff peaks are formed
1 (13.5-ounce) can full-fat coconut milk
1 (13.5-ounce) can coconut cream
¾ cup granulated erythritol–monk
  fruit blend

2 large eggs
2 large egg yolks
2 teaspoons vanilla extract
1 tablespoon unflavored gelatin
1¾ cups unsweetened
  shredded coconut

FOR THE TOPPING

¼ cup unsweetened shredded coconut
2 cups heavy (whipping) cream
¼ cup granulated erythritol–monk
  fruit blend
1 ounce full-fat cream cheese, at room
  temperature

TO MAKE THE CRUST

1. Preheat the oven to 360°F. Grease the pie dish with butter and set aside.

2. In a large bowl, combine the coconut flour, melted butter, eggs, erythritol–monk fruit blend, and salt. Mix just until the dough forms. Pat and press the crust into the bottom and sides of the prepared pie dish. Bake for 15 minutes, until lightly browned. Set on the cooling rack to cool, 15 to 20 minutes.

TO MAKE THE FILLING

3. In the saucepan, bring the heavy cream, coconut milk, coconut cream, erythritol–monk fruit blend, whole eggs, egg yolks, and vanilla to a slow simmer over medium heat. Continue to stir, being careful not to let the mixture come to a boil. Once the mixture comes to a slow simmer, sprinkle with the gelatin while whisking constantly. Add the shredded coconut and continue to mix, cooking the filling for 5 to 7 minutes, until it starts to thicken.

4. Allow the mixture to cool for about 10 minutes before adding it to the prepared crust. Refrigerate the pie until chilled, about 4 hours.

TO MAKE THE TOPPING

5. While the pie chills, in the medium skillet, toast the coconut over medium-low heat for 3 to 5 minutes, until lightly browned. Remove from the skillet and set aside.

6. In another large bowl, using an electric mixer on high, whip the heavy cream, erythritol–monk fruit blend, and cream cheese for 3 to 5 minutes, until stiff peaks form. Top the chilled pie with the whipped cream and sprinkle with the toasted coconut. Cut into 10 slices and serve.

7. Store leftovers in an airtight container in the refrigerator for up to 5 days.

KEEP IN MIND: The filling mixture will continue to thicken once it is allowed to chill completely, so don't fret if it seems too thin. Wetting your hands will make it easier to pat the crust in place without sticking to you. Cover the edges of the crust with foil to prevent it from browning too much.

Per serving: Calories: 793; Total Fat: 77g; Total Carbohydrates: 15g; Net Carbs: 8g; Fiber: 7g; Protein: 10g Sweetener: 20g
Macros: Fat: 87%; Protein: 5%; Carbs: 8%

Raspberry Mousse Tart

PREP TIME: 15 minutes **COOK TIME:** 45 minutes, plus 35 minutes to cool **CHILL TIME:** 20 minutes
EQUIPMENT: 2 small mixing bowls, large mixing bowl, medium glass mixing bowl, spatula, electric mixer, small saucepan, 9-inch tart pan with removable bottom, sieve, cooling rack

Bust out this tart for your next celebration! A raspberry-infused lemon curd takes this concoction to the next level.

FOR THE CURD

8 tablespoons (1 stick) unsalted butter, at room temperature

5 cups fresh or frozen raspberries, plus more for garnish

1 cup granulated erythritol–monk fruit blend

¼ cup freshly squeezed lemon juice

¼ teaspoon sea salt

6 large egg yolks

FOR THE CRUST

4 tablespoons (½ stick) unsalted butter, melted, plus more for greasing

1½ cups finely milled almond flour, sifted

¼ cup granulated erythritol–monk fruit blend

2 tablespoons freshly squeezed lemon juice

¼ teaspoon sea salt

FOR THE MOUSSE

6 tablespoons cold water

2 teaspoons unflavored gelatin

16 ounces full-fat cream cheese

1 cup granulated erythritol–monk fruit blend

1 cup full-fat sour cream

¼ teaspoon sea salt

1 cup heavy (whipping) cream

TO MAKE THE CURD

1. In the small saucepan, bring 1 inch of water to a boil over medium-high heat. Set the glass mixing bowl over the saucepan (but not touching the water). Add the butter to the bowl. Once melted, add the raspberries, erythritol–monk fruit blend, lemon juice, and salt. Stir frequently, mashing the berries. Reduce the heat to low and add the egg yolks one at a time, whisking quickly.

2. Whisk constantly while cooking for 7 to 10 minutes, until the curd thickens. Remove the curd from the heat and strain through the sieve, mashing the berries with a spoon. Allow the curd to fully cool at room temperature, about 15 minutes.

TO MAKE THE CRUST

3. Preheat the oven to 350°F. Grease the tart pan with butter and set aside.

4. In a small bowl, combine the almond flour, granulated erythritol–monk fruit blend, lemon juice, and salt. Add the melted butter and combine well.

5. Press the mixture into the tart pan. Bake for 20 to 25 minutes, until lightly browned. Cool on the cooling rack, about 20 minutes.

TO MAKE THE MOUSSE

6. In another small bowl, mix together the cold water and unflavored gelatin and set aside.

7. In the large bowl, using an electric mixer on high, beat the cream cheese, granulated erythritol–monk fruit blend, sour cream, mixed gelatin, and salt until fully combined. Be sure to scrape the sides of the bowl several times. Slowly add in the heavy cream.

8. Once the curd has fully cooled, gently fold it into the cream cheese mixture until fully combined. Put in the refrigerator for about 20 minutes while the crust fully cools.

9. To assemble the tart, spoon the curd-mousse mixture into the tart shell, using a spatula to spread the mixture evenly. Put the tart pan on an upturned jar or glass on the counter and gently slide the ring from the bottom of the tart pan down. Lift the tart off and carefully slide it off the bottom of the pan and onto a serving plate. Garnish with the reserved raspberries.

VARIATION TIP: Make tartlets in 5 (4-inch) tart pans and reduce baking time by 10 to 15 minutes.

Per serving: Calories: 569; Total Fat: 53g; Total Carbohydrates: 14g; Net Carbs: 8g; Fiber: 6g; Protein: 9g; Sweetener: 43g
Macros: Fat: 84%; Protein: 6%; Carbs: 10%

Lemon Curd Tartlets

PREP TIME: 15 minutes **COOK TIME:** 35 minutes, plus 35 minutes to cool **CHILL TIME:** 20 minutes
EQUIPMENT: 2 small mixing bowls, large mixing bowl, large glass mixing bowl, electric mixer, small saucepan, 5 (4-inch) tart pans

A rich buttery crust filled with the smoothest, tangiest lemon curd filling makes these tartlets a delectable dessert for a summer barbecue. The cool lemon and light and airy mousse satisfy your sweet tooth without weighing you down.

TO MAKE THE CURD

4 tablespoons (½ stick) unsalted butter, at room temperature

7 large egg yolks

¾ cup granulated erythritol–monk fruit blend

1 tablespoon grated lemon zest

¾ cup freshly squeezed lemon juice (about 3 large lemons)

½ teaspoon lemon extract

¼ teaspoon sea salt

FOR THE CRUST

4 tablespoons (½ stick) unsalted butter, melted, plus more for greasing

1½ cups finely milled almond flour, sifted

¼ cup granulated erythritol–monk fruit blend

2 tablespoons freshly squeezed lemon juice

¼ teaspoon sea salt

FOR THE MOUSSE

6 tablespoons cold water

2 teaspoons unflavored gelatin

16 ounces full-fat cream cheese

1 cup full-fat sour cream

1 cup granulated erythritol–monk fruit blend

½ teaspoon lemon extract

½ teaspoon grated lemon zest

¼ teaspoon sea salt

1 cup heavy (whipping) cream

TO MAKE THE CURD

1. In the small saucepan, bring 1 inch of water to a boil over medium-high heat. Set the glass mixing bowl over the saucepan (without touching the water). Add the butter to the bowl. Once melted, add the egg yolks, one at a time, whisking quickly. Add the erythritol–monk fruit blend, lemon zest, lemon juice, lemon extract, and salt.

2. Whisk constantly while cooking for 7 to 10 minutes, until the mixture thickens. Remove from the heat and allow the curd to fully cool at room temperature, about 15 minutes.

TO MAKE THE CRUST

3. Preheat the oven to 350°F. Grease the tart pans with butter.

4. In a small bowl, combine the almond flour, erythritol–monk fruit blend, lemon juice, and salt. Add the melted butter and combine well. Spread the mixture evenly among the tart pans and press into their bottoms and sides.

5. Bake for 10 to 15 minutes, until lightly browned, and cool for 15 to 20 minutes.

TO MAKE THE MOUSSE

6. In another small bowl, mix together the cold water and gelatin and set aside.

7. In the large bowl, using an electric mixer on high, beat the cream cheese, sour cream, erythritol–monk fruit blend, softened gelatin, lemon extract, lemon zest, and salt until fully combined. Slowly add the heavy cream. Refrigerate until all parts are chilled, about 20 minutes.

8. Assemble the tarts by spreading the mousse mixture in the tart shells and topping with the curd. Chill the assembled tarts in the refrigerator for 15 minutes.

9. To unmold, put one tart pan on an upturned small glass on the counter and gently slide the ring from the bottom of the tart pan down the glass. Lift the tart off and carefully slide it off the bottom of the pan and onto a serving plate. Repeat with the remaining tart pans and serve.

10. Store leftovers in an airtight container in the refrigerator for up to 3 days.

SPICE IT UP: Garnish these tarts with fresh blueberries!

Per serving: Calories: 980; Total Fat: 97g; Total Carbohydrates: 16g; Net Carbs: 12g; Fiber: 4g; Protein: 18g; Sweetener: 77g
Macros: Fat: 86%; Protein: 8%; Carbs: 6%

Cinnamon Pecan "Apple" Crisp

PREP TIME: 20 minutes **COOK TIME:** 1 hour 20 minutes, plus 20 minutes to cool
EQUIPMENT: 2 medium mixing bowls, medium saucepan, 9-by-9-inch baking pan

When you're craving homestyle comfort food, this easy "apple" crisp delivers. Made with sliced chayote squash and a crispy streusel topping, it's perfectly keto. Bonus: You don't have to fuss with making and rolling out pie dough.

FOR THE FILLING

2 tablespoons unsalted butter, chilled and sliced, plus more for greasing

4 chayote squash

¾ cup granulated erythritol–monk fruit blend; *less sweet:* ½ cup

½ cup freshly squeezed lemon juice

2 tablespoons ground cinnamon

½ teaspoon ground ginger

½ teaspoon cream of tartar

¼ teaspoon ground nutmeg

FOR THE TOPPING

1½ cups finely milled almond flour, sifted

½ cup coconut flour

3 tablespoons granulated erythritol–monk fruit blend

1 teaspoon baking powder

¼ teaspoon sea salt

4 tablespoons (½ stick) unsalted butter, chilled and sliced

½ cup pecan halves

2 tablespoons ground cinnamon

2 large eggs, at room temperature

TO MAKE THE FILLING

1. Preheat the oven to 350°F. Grease the baking pan with butter and set aside.

2. In the medium saucepan, cover the chayote squash with water and boil for 25 to 30 minutes. They should be firm but cooked through. Allow the squash to cool, 15 to 20 minutes, then peel and cut into ¼-inch-thick slices.

3. In a medium bowl, combine the squash, erythritol–monk fruit blend, lemon juice, cinnamon, ginger, cream of tartar, and nutmeg. Combine well.

4. Add the filling to the prepared pan and dot with the sliced butter.

TO MAKE THE TOPPING

5. In another medium bowl, combine the almond flour, coconut flour, erythritol–monk fruit blend, baking powder, and salt. Add the butter and mix until crumbly and resembling coarse cornmeal. Stir in the pecans and cinnamon. Add the eggs and combine well, but do not overmix.

6. Spoon the topping over the filling in the baking pan, being sure to break up larger pieces, and distribute evenly. Bake for 35 to 40 minutes, until hot and bubbling. Cut into 12 pieces and serve warm or cold.

7. Store leftovers in an airtight container in the refrigerator for up to 5 days.

VARIATION TIP: If you are unable to find chayote squash, you could use peeled and chopped zucchini instead and reduce boiling time to 3 to 5 minutes, or until slightly tender.

Per serving: Calories: 206; Total Fat: 18g; Total Carbohydrates: 10g; Net Carbs: 5g; Fiber: 5g; Protein: 6g; Sweetener: 16g
Macros: Fat: 74%; Protein: 9%; Carbs: 17%

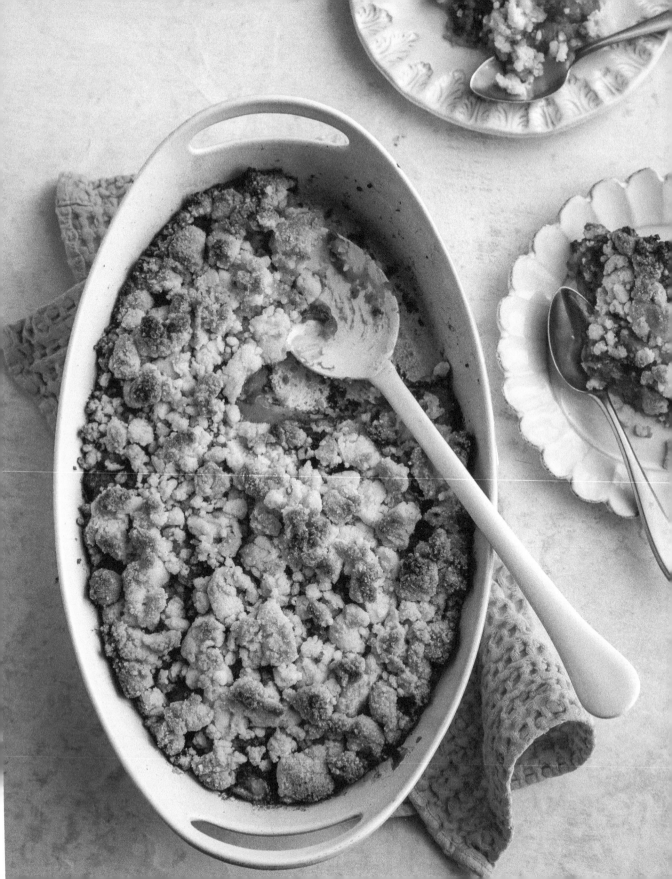

Mixed Berry Crisp

PREP TIME: 20 minutes **COOK TIME:** 40 minutes
EQUIPMENT: large mixing bowl, medium mixing bowl, 8-by-8-inch baking pan

Strawberries, raspberries, and blueberries under a perfectly crisp crust. Need I say more? Sometimes I like to switch up the presentation and bake this in a ceramic baking dish, or even individual ramekins.

FOR THE TOPPING

8 tablespoons (1 stick) unsalted butter, chilled and sliced, plus more for greasing

2 cups finely milled almond flour

½ cup granulated erythritol–monk fruit blend; *less sweet: ¼ cup*

1 teaspoon baking powder

¼ teaspoon sea salt

1 large egg, lightly beaten

FOR THE FILLING

1 cup sliced fresh or frozen strawberries

½ cup fresh or frozen blueberries

½ cup fresh or frozen raspberries

¼ cup granulated erythritol–monk fruit blend; *less sweet: 3 tablespoons*

¼ teaspoon xanthan gum

TO MAKE THE TOPPING

1. Preheat the oven to 350°F. Grease the baking pan with butter and set aside.

2. In the large bowl, combine the almond flour, erythritol–monk fruit blend, baking powder, and salt and mix well. Mix in the butter with a fork until the pieces are pea-size. Mix in the egg until well combined. Press half the topping into the baking pan.

TO MAKE THE FILLING

3. In the medium bowl, mix the berries, erythritol–monk fruit blend, and xanthan gum.

4. Spread the fruit in the pan and cover with the remaining topping. Bake for 40 minutes, until the top is golden brown. Serve warm or cold.

5. Store leftovers in an airtight container in the refrigerator for up to 5 days.

Per serving: Calories: 176; **Total Fat:** 16g; **Total Carbohydrates:** 6g; **Net Carbs:** 3g; **Fiber:** 3g; **Protein:** 4g; **Sweetener:** 12g
Macros: Fat: 78%; **Protein:** 9%; **Carbs:** 13%

Blueberry Crumble

PREP TIME: 10 minutes COOK TIME: 40 minutes, plus 20 minutes to cool
EQUIPMENT: large mixing bowl, medium mixing bowl, 9-by-13-inch baking sheet

This Southern favorite made keto is everything you want in a summer dessert. In the fall, substitute the "apple" pie mixture from the "Apple" Pie (page 128) for the filling.

FOR THE TOPPING

3½ cups finely milled almond flour

1 cup granulated erythritol–monk fruit blend

1½ teaspoons baking powder

½ teaspoon sea salt

1 cup (2 sticks) unsalted butter, chilled and sliced, plus more for greasing

1 large egg, lightly beaten

FOR THE FILLING

4 cups blueberries

½ cup granulated erythritol–monk fruit blend

3 tablespoons freshly squeezed lemon juice

½ teaspoon xanthan gum

TO MAKE THE TOPPING

1. In the large bowl, combine the almond flour, erythritol–monk fruit blend, baking powder, and salt. Add the butter and use a fork to mix until the pieces are pea-size. Add the beaten egg and continue to mix until well combined. Set aside.

TO MAKE THE FILLING

2. Preheat the oven to 350°F. Grease the baking sheet with butter and set aside.

3. In the medium bowl, mix together the blueberries, erythritol–monk fruit blend, lemon juice, and xanthan gum.

4. Spoon the blueberry mixture into the baking sheet and cover with the topping.

5. Bake for 40 minutes, until the top is golden brown. Allow the crumble to cool slightly, 15 to 20 minutes, then cut into 15 pieces and serve.

6. Store leftovers in an airtight container in the refrigerator for up to 5 days.

Per serving: Calories: 265; Total Fat: 24g; Total Carbohydrates: 11g; Net Carbs: 7g; Fiber: 4g; Protein: 6g; Sweetener: 19g
Macros: Fat: 77%; Protein: 9%; Carbs: 14%

Strawberry Rhubarb Cobbler

SERVES 15

PREP TIME: 15 minutes **COOK TIME:** 40 minutes, plus 10 minutes to cool
EQUIPMENT: large mixing bowl, medium mixing bowl, 9-by-13-inch baking sheet

Cobbler makes a fantastic finale to any meal. Cut leftovers into rectangles to make cobbler bars that you can refrigerate for up to 5 days

FOR THE TOPPING

1 cup (2 sticks) unsalted butter, chilled
   and sliced, plus more for greasing
3½ cups finely milled almond flour
1 cup granulated erythritol–monk
   fruit blend
1½ teaspoons baking powder
½ teaspoon sea salt
1 large egg, lightly beaten

FOR THE FILLING

3 cups sliced fresh or frozen
   strawberries
2 cups sliced fresh or frozen rhubarb
½ cup granulated erythritol–monk
   fruit blend
½ teaspoon xanthan gum

TO MAKE THE TOPPING

1. Preheat the oven to 350°F. Grease the baking sheet with butter and set aside.

2. In the large bowl, combine the almond flour, erythritol–monk fruit blend, baking powder, and salt. Add the butter and use a fork to mix until the pieces are pea-size. Add the beaten egg and continue to mix until well combined.

3. Divide the topping and press half of it into the bottom of the baking sheet.

TO MAKE THE FILLING

4. In the medium bowl, mix together the strawberries, rhubarb, erythritol–monk fruit blend, and xanthan gum.

5. Spoon this mixture on top of the crumb base in the baking sheet, spreading it evenly. Top with the other half of the crumb mixture. Bake for 40 minutes, until the top is golden brown. Allow to cool slightly, 5 to 10 minutes, before serving.

Per serving: Calories: 256; **Total Fat:** 24g; **Total Carbohydrates:** 8g; **Net Carbs:** 4g; **Fiber:** 4g; **Protein:** 6g; Sweetener: 19g
Macros: Fat: 80%; Protein: 8%; Carbs: 12%

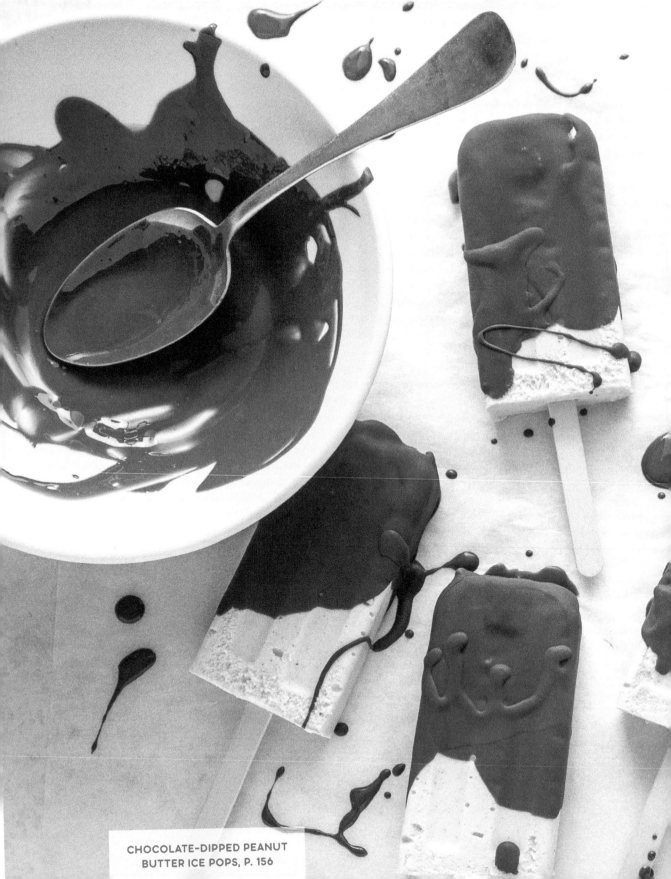

CHOCOLATE-DIPPED PEANUT
BUTTER ICE POPS, P. 156

CHAPTER EIGHT

Drinks and Frozen Treats

PB and J Smoothie 144

Eggnog 145

Salted Hot Chocolate 147

Strawberry Mojito Mocktail Slushie 149

Coffee Granitas 150

Lemon-Lime Granitas 151

Dairy-Free Mocha Ice "Cream" 152

Chocolate-Vanilla Ice Cream Cake 153

Strawberries and Cream Ice Pops 155

Chocolate-Dipped Peanut Butter Ice Pops 156

Dairy-Free Chocolate Fudge Pops 157

PB and J Smoothie

PREP TIME: 5 minutes **COOK TIME:** 5 minutes
EQUIPMENT: blender

If you thought enjoying smoothies was out of the question while on a keto diet, think again. This smoothie uses coconut milk and sour cream in place of yogurt for low-carb creaminess. To save time in the morning, add all of your ingredients, except for the frozen berries and water, to the blender pitcher and put it in the refrigerator.

¾ cup frozen mixed berries (blueberries, raspberries, and blackberries)

¼ cup full-fat sour cream

½ cup full-fat coconut milk

¼ cup water

1½ tablespoons all-natural peanut butter (no added sugar)

½ tablespoon granulated erythritol–monk fruit blend (optional)

In a blender, blend the frozen mixed berries, sour cream, coconut milk, water, peanut butter, and erythritol–monk fruit blend (if using). Pulse a few times to get the ingredients to fall to the bottom, and blend for about 1 minute, or until smooth. If the blender struggles, add a few tablespoons of water and try again. Serve and enjoy immediately.

INGREDIENT TIP: I recommend using frozen berries, but if you prefer fresh, add ¼ cup of ice.

Per serving (1 cup): **Calories:** 266; **Total Fat:** 23g; **Total Carbohydrates:** 11g; **Net Carbs:** 9g; **Fiber:** 2g; **Protein:** 5g; **Sweetener:** 9g
Macros: Fat: 78%; **Protein:** 6%; **Carbs:** 16%

Eggnog

PREP TIME: 5 minutes **COOK TIME:** 30 minutes **CHILL TIME:** 1 hour
EQUIPMENT: 2 medium mixing bowls, electric mixer, medium saucepan, sieve, plastic wrap

Winter holidays are even more festive with low-carb eggnog! I can't imagine celebrating Christmas without it. Make it dairy-free by using coconut cream instead of heavy cream.

1¼ cups almond milk

1 cup heavy (whipping) cream

½ teaspoon ground cinnamon

¼ teaspoon ground nutmeg, plus more for dusting

¼ teaspoon sea salt

4 large egg yolks

½ cup granulated erythritol–monk fruit blend

¼ cup dark rum or 1½ teaspoons rum extract

1 teaspoon vanilla extract

1. In the medium saucepan, heat the almond milk, heavy cream, cinnamon, nutmeg, and salt over medium heat and lightly simmer for about 10 minutes to reduce slightly.

2. In a medium bowl, using an electric mixer on medium, mix the egg yolks and erythritol–monk fruit blend for about 3 minutes, until light and fluffy.

3. Temper the hot mixture into the egg mixture by slowing adding the hot liquid to the egg mixture, whisking constantly to prevent the egg yolks from curdling.

4. Add the mixture back to the saucepan and cook over medium-low heat for about 10 minutes, until it coats the back of a spoon. Remove from the heat and pour through the sieve into another medium bowl. Stir in the rum and vanilla.

5. Cover with plastic wrap and refrigerate until fully chilled, about 1 hour, before serving. Pour into glasses and dust with nutmeg to serve.

6. Store leftovers in an airtight container in the refrigerator for up to 3 days.

KEEP IN MIND: The eggnog will continue to thicken as it cools, so don't be worried if it seems too liquidy when you remove it from the heat.

Per serving (6 ounces): **Calories:** 311; **Total Fat:** 29g; **Total Carbohydrates:** 6g; **Net Carbs:** 6g; **Fiber:** 0g; **Protein:** 6g; **Sweetener:** 24g
Macros: Fat: 83%; **Protein:** 9%; **Carbs:** 8%

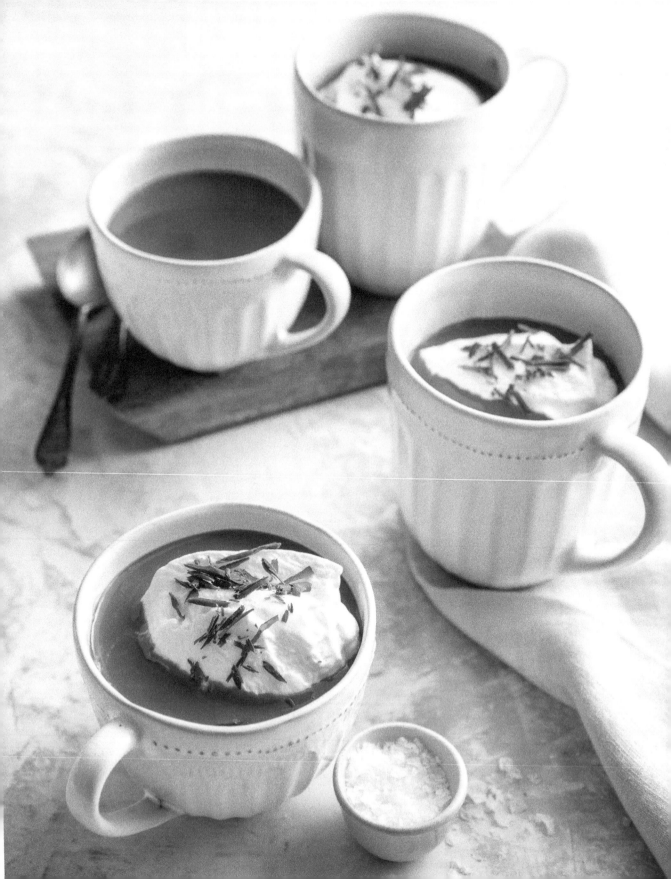

Salted Hot Chocolate

SERVES 4

PREP TIME: 5 minutes **COOK TIME:** 10 minutes
EQUIPMENT: medium saucepan

The moment the temperature drops, you'll want to reach for this salted hot chocolate. I like curling up on the couch with a mug of this and a good movie on cold nights. Don't hesitate to top it with some keto-friendly whipped cream and a few shavings of dark chocolate. If you're using coconut milk, make sure you get coconut milk beverage, which comes in cartons, not the coconut milk in cans, which will be too thick for this.

6 tablespoons granulated erythritol–monk fruit blend; *less sweet:* *4 tablespoons*

¼ cup unsweetened cocoa powder

½ cup heavy (whipping) cream (or coconut cream for a dairy-free option)

2 cups unsweetened almond or coconut milk beverage

1 teaspoon vanilla extract

¼ teaspoon sea salt

1. In the saucepan, not over heat, whisk the erythritol–monk fruit blend and cocoa powder until there are no visible lumps.

2. Set the saucepan over low heat and slowly pour in the heavy cream, a little bit at a time, while stirring constantly, until a thick sauce has formed. Slowly whisk in the almond milk and increase the heat to medium-low until the mixture is heated through, taking care not to let the hot chocolate boil.

3. Remove the pan from the heat and stir in the vanilla and salt. Serve immediately in mugs.

4. Store leftovers in an airtight container in the refrigerator for up to 3 days.

KEEP IN MIND: The hot chocolate can be reheated, but do so in a saucepan over low heat rather than in a microwave to ensure even heating and to prevent burning.

Per serving (5¼ ounces): Calories: 393; **Total Fat:** 40g; **Total Carbohydrates:** 10g; **Net Carbs:** 6g; **Fiber:** 4g; **Protein:** 4g; **Sweetener:** 18g
Macros: Fat: 87%; **Protein:** 4%; **Carbs:** 9%

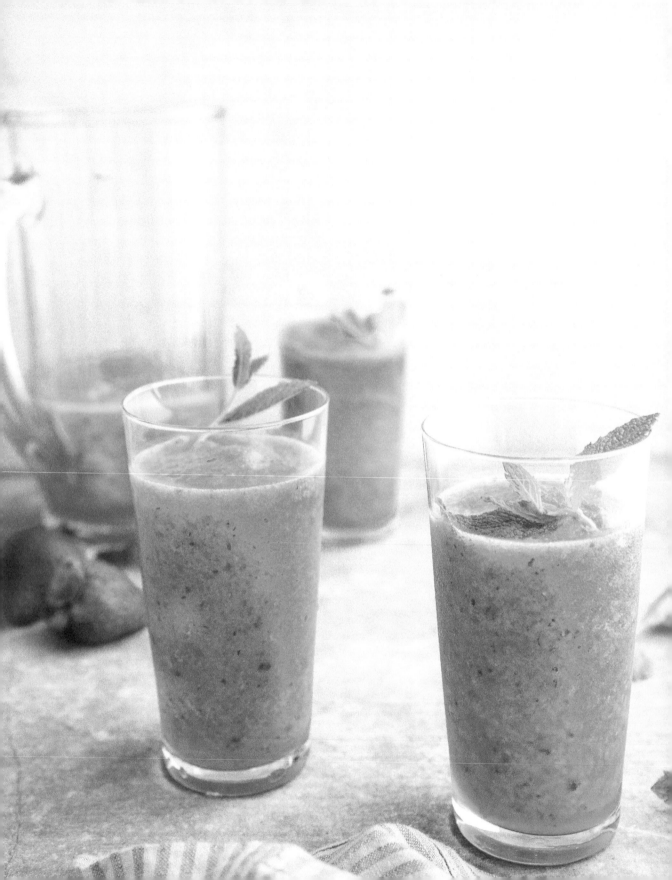

Strawberry Mojito Mocktail Slushie

PREP TIME: 10 minutes **COOK TIME:** 5 minutes
EQUIPMENT: blender, small saucepan

This slushie will become your new go-to for summer parties. To make it boozy, add ½ cup of clear rum along with the lime juice.

FOR THE LIME SIMPLE SYRUP

½ cup water
½ cup granulated erythritol–monk fruit blend
1½ teaspoons grated lime zest

FOR THE MOJITO MOCKTAIL

1 cup chopped fresh or frozen strawberries
5 cups ice
¼ cup freshly squeezed lime juice
1 tablespoon coarsely chopped fresh mint
6 mint sprigs, for garnish

TO MAKE THE LIME SIMPLE SYRUP

1. In the saucepan, heat the water, erythritol–monk fruit blend, and lime zest over low heat until the erythritol–monk fruit blend dissolves, whisking occasionally. Set aside.

TO MAKE THE MOJITO MOCKTAIL

2. In a blender, combine the strawberries and 1 tablespoon of the lime simple syrup and pulse until the strawberries are pureed. Add the ice, remaining syrup, and lime juice. Blend until the ice is crushed. Add the chopped mint and blend until the mixture is completely blended.

3. Garnish with a mint sprig and serve immediately in a tall glass.

VARIATION TIP: Leave out the lime zest for a simple syrup to use in a variety of cocktails and mocktails. Or, simmer a chunk of ginger in the syrup for a Moscow Mule!

Per serving (1 cup): Calories: 11; Total Fat: 0g; Total Carbohydrates: 3g; Net Carbs: 2g; Fiber: 1g; Protein: 0g; Sweetener: 16g
Macros: Fat: 6%; Protein: 7%; Carbs: 87%

Coffee Granitas

PREP TIME: 10 minutes **CHILL TIME:** 3 hours
EQUIPMENT: blender, 9-by-5-inch loaf pan

This coffee granita is like a snow cone for grown-ups! Leftovers won't keep (they will freeze solid), so invite your friends over to enjoy this treat with you.

4 cups strongly brewed coffee, cooled

3 tablespoons granulated erythritol–monk fruit blend; *less sweet:*
1 tablespoon

1¼ teaspoons vanilla extract

Whipped cream, for serving (optional)

1. In a blender (or in a large bowl with an electric mixer on high), whisk together the coffee, erythritol–monk fruit blend, and vanilla until the color of the coffee turns light in color and foamy, almost like a cappuccino.

2. Pour the coffee mixture into the loaf pan and put in the freezer for 1 hour. After the hour, stir and scrape the mixture with a fork and put back in the freezer. Repeat every 30 minutes for 2 to 3 hours, until the mixture is semi-frozen and resembles snow.

3. Serve in small glasses with whipped cream (if using) on the bottom of the glass as well as on the top.

KEEP IN MIND: It's key to wait for the coffee to be completely cooled before mixing and freezing or it will take a very long time to freeze and might not reach the snow consistency.

Per serving (1 cup): Calories: 6; Total Fat: 0g; Total Carbohydrates: 0g; Net Carbs: 0g; Fiber: 0g; Protein: 0g; Sweetener: 12g
Macros: Fat: 20%; Protein: 48%; Carbs: 32%

Lemon-Lime Granitas

PREP TIME: 15 minutes **COOK TIME:** 5 minutes, plus 20 minutes to cool **CHILL TIME:** 3 hours
EQUIPMENT: small saucepan, 9-by-5-inch loaf pan

On a hot summer day, nothing is quite as refreshing as a glass of lemonade—except for this lemon-lime granita. The addition of lime juice and citrus zest elevates this frosty treat. Leftovers will freeze solid, so enjoy these granitas right away.

4 cups water

¾ cup granulated erythritol–monk fruit blend; *less sweet: ½ cup*

1 teaspoon grated lemon zest

1 teaspoon grated lime zest

⅓ cup freshly squeezed lemon juice

⅓ cup freshly squeezed lime juice

1. In the saucepan, heat the water, erythritol–monk fruit blend, lemon zest, lime zest, lemon juice, and lime juice over low heat. Stir occasionally until the erythritol–monk fruit blend has dissolved. Set aside and let cool completely, 15 to 20 minutes.

2. Pour the cooled mixture into the loaf pan and put in the freezer for 1 hour. After the hour, stir and scrape the mixture with a fork. Repeat every 30 minutes for 2 to 3 hours, until the mixture is semi-frozen and resembles snow. Serve in small glasses and enjoy immediately.

VARIATION TIP: For a different flavor, add 1 teaspoon of finely chopped ginger in step 1 while heating. You could also try adding mint to make mock mojito granitas.

Per serving (1 cup): Calories: 9; Total Fat: 0g; Total Carbohydrates: 2g; Net Carbs: 2g; Fiber: 0g; Protein: 0g; Sweetener: 36g
Macros: Fat: 6%; Protein: 5%; Carbs: 89%

Dairy-Free Mocha Ice "Cream"

PREP TIME: 5 minutes **CHILL TIME:** 2 hours
EQUIPMENT: large mixing bowl, electric mixer, 2 (9-by-5-inch) loaf pans, parchment paper

This rich and creamy chocolate ice cream made with coconut milk requires virtually zero effort and no specialized equipment. Because it's dairy-free, anyone can enjoy it.

4 (13.5-ounce) cans full-fat coconut milk, chilled overnight

1 cup granulated erythritol–monk fruit blend; *less sweet: ½ cup*

6 tablespoons unsweetened cocoa powder

2 teaspoons instant espresso powder

½ teaspoon sea salt

1. Line the loaf pans with parchment paper and set aside.

2. In the large bowl, using an electric mixer on low, mix the coconut milk, erythritol–monk fruit blend, cocoa powder, espresso, and salt for 1 to 2 minutes, until fully combined, stopping and scraping the sides once or twice, as needed.

3. Pour the mixture into the prepared loaf pans and freeze solid, about 2 hours.

4. Allow to soften on the counter for a few minutes before enjoying.

5. Store in the freezer for up to 3 weeks.

KEEP IN MIND: A blender works just as well as an electric mixer for this recipe. For a creamier version, stir the ice cream with a fork every 30 minutes to break up the ice from the coconut milk as it freezes to create a smoother texture. Serve as soon as it is frozen to your liking.

Per serving (⅓ cup): **Calories:** 193; **Total Fat:** 21g; **Total Carbohydrates:** 4g; **Net Carbs:** 3g; **Fiber:** 1g;
Protein: 2g; **Sweetener:** 12g
Macros: Fat: 89%; **Protein:** 4%; **Carbs:** 9%

Chocolate-Vanilla Ice Cream Cake

SERVES 16

PREP TIME: 15 minutes **COOK TIME:** 45 minutes, plus 20 minutes to cool **CHILL TIME:** 4 hours
EQUIPMENT: 2 small mixing bowls, 2 large mixing bowls, electric mixer, small microwave-safe bowl,
2 (9-inch) round cake pans, 10-by-10-inch freezer-safe baking pan, toothpicks

Birthdays beg to be celebrated with ice cream cake. This low-carb, sugar-free alternative is endlessly adaptable. You can use any keto cake, like the Brown Butter Bundt Cake recipe on page 88.

FOR THE CAKE

4 tablespoons (½ stick) unsalted butter, melted, plus more for greasing

½ cup heavy (whipping) cream

½ cup cold water

2 cups granulated erythritol–monk fruit blend

1 cup finely milled almond flour, sifted

¾ cup coconut flour

¾ cup unsweetened cocoa powder

1½ teaspoons baking powder

1½ teaspoons baking soda

½ teaspoon sea salt

3 large eggs

2 teaspoons vanilla extract

1 cup boiling water

FOR THE ICE CREAM LAYER

8 ounces full-fat cream cheese, at room temperature

¾ cup confectioners' erythritol–monk fruit blend

1 teaspoon vanilla extract

¼ teaspoon sea salt

2 cups heavy (whipping) cream, cold

FOR THE CHOCOLATE SAUCE TOPPING

3 tablespoons coconut oil, melted

3 tablespoons confectioners' erythritol–monk fruit blend

2 teaspoons unsweetened cocoa powder

¼ teaspoon sea salt

TO MAKE THE CAKE

1. Preheat the oven to 350°F. Grease the cake pans with butter.

2. In a small bowl, combine the heavy cream and cold water.

3. In a large bowl, combine the granulated erythritol–monk fruit blend, almond flour, coconut flour, cocoa powder, baking powder, baking soda, and salt. To the dry ingredients, using an electric mixer on medium, add the eggs, heavy cream mixture, melted butter, and vanilla, and mix until combined. Add the boiling water and stir until well blended.

4. Pour the batter into the two prepared cake pans and bake for 35 to 45 minutes, or until a toothpick inserted into the center comes out clean. Once the cakes have cooled, 15 to 20 minutes, crumble and evenly divide into two parts. Press half the cake crumbs into the bottom of the freezer-safe baking pan.

TO MAKE THE ICE CREAM LAYER

5. In another large bowl, using an electric mixer on high, mix the cream cheese, confectioners' erythritol–monk fruit blend, vanilla, and salt. Mix at high speed, scraping the sides of the bowl a few times. Once combined, add the heavy cream a little at a time, continuing to mix until it is fully incorporated into the cream cheese mixture.

6. Pour the ice cream mixture on top of the layer of cake crumbs in the baking pan and spread evenly. Add the remaining cake crumbs directly over the ice cream and gently press the crumbs into the surface of the mixture. Transfer the ice cream cake to the freezer for at least 4 hours or until it is frozen solid.

TO MAKE THE CHOCOLATE SAUCE TOPPING

7. Once the cake is frozen, in another small bowl, combine the melted coconut oil, confectioners' erythritol–monk fruit blend, cocoa powder, and salt. Drizzle the chocolate sauce over the cake. The topping will quickly harden, and the cake is ready to be served immediately.

8. Store leftovers in an airtight container in the freezer for up to 2 weeks.

VARIATION TIP: Can't get enough chocolate? Add ¾ cup of cocoa powder to the ice cream mixture to make this a chocolate-on-chocolate ice cream cake.

Per serving: Calories: 301; Total Fat: 30g; Total Carbohydrates: 6g; Net Carbs: 3g; Fiber: 3g; Protein: 5g; Sweetener: 35g
Macros: Fat: 87%; Protein: 6%; Carbs: 7%

Strawberries and Cream Ice Pops

MAKES 12

PREP TIME: 10 minutes **CHILL TIME:** 4 hours
EQUIPMENT: blender, 12 popsicle molds

These refreshing strawberries and cream ice pops are best made with a blender, but a food processor or electric mixer will work, too. These taste so delicious, you won't believe they only take 10 minutes to prepare.

2 cups heavy (whipping) cream

8 ounces full-fat cream cheese, at room temperature

¼ cup full-fat sour cream

1 tablespoon freshly squeezed lemon juice

1½ cups sliced strawberries, divided

1 cup blueberries, divided

¾ cup granulated erythritol–monk fruit blend; *less sweet: ½ cup*

1. In a blender, combine the heavy cream, cream cheese, sour cream, and lemon juice and blend until smooth. Add 1 cup of strawberries, ½ cup of blueberries, and the erythritol–monk fruit blend and blend until fully combined and smooth.

2. Spoon the remaining berries into each popsicle mold, then pour the cream mixture into each mold. Add the popsicle sticks. Freeze for 3 to 4 hours, until frozen solid. Serve immediately after unmolding.

3. Store in the freezer in an airtight container for up to 3 weeks.

VARIATION TIP: Make orange cream ice pops instead by omitting the berries and adding 1 teaspoon of orange extract. This will make fewer popsicles, however.

Per serving (1 pop): **Calories:** 225: **Total Fat:** 22g: **Total Carbohydrates:** 6g: **Net Carbs:** 5g: **Fiber:** 1g: **Protein:** 2g: **Sweetener:** 12g
Macros: Fat: 87%: **Protein:** 4%: **Carbs:** 9%

Chocolate-Dipped
Peanut Butter Ice Pops

MAKES 12

PREP TIME: 10 minutes **COOK TIME:** 5 minutes **CHILL TIME:** 4 hours
EQUIPMENT: large mixing bowl, electric mixer, small microwave-safe bowl, 12-by-17-inch baking sheet, 12 popsicle molds

These smooth and creamy ice pops are perfect for those who find the classic combination of peanut butter and chocolate absolutely irresistible.

8 ounces full-fat cream cheese, at room temperature

1 cup all-natural peanut butter (no added sugar or salt)

¼ cup confectioners' erythritol–monk fruit blend; *less sweet: 2 tablespoons*

1 teaspoon vanilla extract

¼ teaspoon sea salt

2 cups heavy (whipping) cream

4 ounces sugar-free chocolate chips

2 tablespoons coconut oil

1. In the large bowl, using an electric mixer on medium high, beat the cream cheese, peanut butter, confectioners' erythritol–monk fruit blend, vanilla, and salt. Add the heavy cream and combine until well incorporated.

2. Pour the mixture into the popsicle molds and add the popsicle sticks. Freeze for 3 to 4 hours, until frozen solid.

3. In the microwave-safe bowl, melt the chocolate baking chips and coconut oil in the microwave in 30-second intervals. Cool for 5 to 10 minutes.

4. Line the baking sheet with parchment paper. Dip the unmolded pops halfway into the melted chocolate, then place them on the prepared sheet and return them to the freezer for about 20 minutes. Store in the freezer in an airtight (nonglass) container for up to 3 weeks.

Per serving (1 pop): **Calories:** 405; **Total Fat:** 37g; **Total Carbohydrates:** 9g; **Net Carbs:** 6g; **Fiber:** 3g; **Protein:** 9g; **Sweetener:** 4g
Macros: Fat: 82%; **Protein:** 9%; **Carbs:** 9%

Dairy-Free Chocolate Fudge Pops

MAKES 12

PREP TIME: 5 minutes **COOK TIME:** 10 minutes, plus 15 minutes to cool **CHILL TIME:** 4 hours
EQUIPMENT: medium saucepan, 12 popsicle molds

You'll be 100 percent ready for summer with these super-simple, homemade chocolate fudge pops. They are better than any high-carb store-bought version—and they're dairy-free, too!

1 cup coconut cream

1 cup coconut milk beverage or almond milk

⅓ cup granulated erythritol–monk fruit blend

¼ cup unsweetened cocoa powder

1 teaspoon vanilla extract

¼ teaspoon xanthan gum

1. In the saucepan, combine the coconut cream, coconut milk, erythritol–monk fruit blend, and cocoa powder and whisk constantly over medium-high heat until it comes to a boil.

2. Remove from the heat and stir in the vanilla. Add the xanthan gum while whisking quickly to combine. Allow the mixture to cool for 15 minutes before pouring into the popsicle molds. Insert the popsicle sticks. Freeze for at least 4 hours, or until solid.

3. Store in the freezer for up to 3 weeks.

KEEP IN MIND: To make the ice pops easier to unmold, run the bottoms of the molds under warm water and jiggle the stick gently before removing them.

Per serving (1 pop): Calories: 108; **Total Fat:** 11g; **Total Carbohydrates:** 3g; **Net Carbs:** 2g; **Fiber:** 1g; **Protein:** 1g; Sweetener: 5g
Macros: Fat: 87%; **Protein:** 4%; **Carbs:** 9%

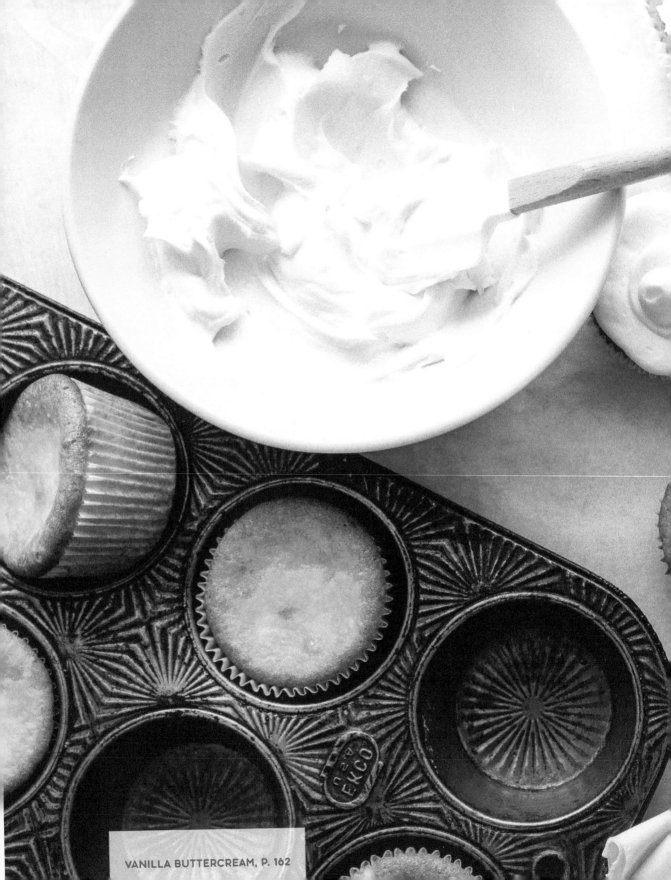

VANILLA BUTTERCREAM, P. 162

CHAPTER NINE

Frostings, Toppings, Sauces, Oh My!

Cream Cheese Frosting 160

Peanut Butter Frosting 161

Vanilla Buttercream 162

Mocha Buttercream 163

Chocolate Ganache 164

Lemon Glaze 165

Dairy-Free Vanilla Icing 166

Whipped Cream 167

Raspberry Sauce 168

Brown Butter Rum Sauce 169

Cream Cheese Frosting

PREP TIME: 10 minutes
EQUIPMENT: large mixing bowl, electric mixer

Creamy, smooth, slightly tangy, and rich, this cream cheese frosting is especially delicious on pumpkin bread and carrot cake. Or spread it on any dessert that calls for icing.

12 ounces full-fat cream cheese, at room temperature

12 tablespoons (1½ sticks) unsalted butter, at room temperature

1 teaspoon vanilla extract

1¼ cups confectioners' erythritol–monk fruit blend

¾ cup heavy (whipping) cream

1. In the large bowl, using an electric mixer on high, beat the cream cheese, butter, and vanilla for 2 to 3 minutes, until light and fluffy. Scrape the sides of the bowl several times as you go. Add the confectioners' erythritol–monk fruit blend a little at a time. Add the heavy cream, a couple of tablespoons at a time, until light and airy, about 2 minutes.

2. Store leftovers in an airtight container in the refrigerator for up to 5 days.

KEEP IN MIND: Make sure your butter and cream cheese are at room temperature. If either is too cold, you won't be able to achieve the light and airy texture we all love in our frostings.

Per serving (2 tablespoons): **Calories:** 94; **Total Fat:** 10g; **Total Carbohydrates:** 1g; **Net Carbs:** 1g; **Fiber:** 0g; **Protein:** 1g; **Sweetener:** 7.5g
Macros: Fat: 94%; **Protein:** 3%; **Carbs:** 3%

Peanut Butter Frosting

MAKES 4 CUPS

PREP TIME: 5 minutes **COOK TIME:** 5 to 10 minutes
EQUIPMENT: large mixing bowl, electric mixer

This creamy, nutty frosting makes a novel topping for cakes and cupcakes. Especially wonderful with chocolate goodies, this frosting gives a lightness to that peanut butter taste.

8 ounces full-fat cream cheese, at room temperature

1 cup all-natural peanut butter (no added sugar or salt)

½ cup confectioners' erythritol–monk fruit blend; *less sweet: ⅓ cup*

4 tablespoons (½ stick) unsalted butter, at room temperature

1 teaspoon vanilla extract

¾ cup heavy (whipping) cream

1. In the large bowl, using an electric mixer on high, mix the cream cheese, peanut butter, confectioners' erythritol–monk fruit blend, butter, and vanilla until well incorporated. With the mixer on, slowly whisk in the heavy cream, until well combined.

2. Store leftovers in an airtight container in the refrigerator for up to 5 days.

KEEP IN MIND: This recipe makes a large amount for the frosting lovers but can easily be halved. It's normal for the frosting to become a bit harder when stored in the refrigerator. To soften it back to its original texture, add a couple of tablespoons of heavy cream.

Per serving (2 tablespoons): Calories: 105; **Total Fat:** 10g; **Total Carbohydrates:** 2g; **Net Carbs:** 2g; **Fiber:** 0g; **Protein:** 2g; **Sweetener:** 3g
Macros: Fat: 83%; **Protein:** 8%; **Carbs:** 9%

Vanilla Buttercream

PREP TIME: 10 minutes
EQUIPMENT: large mixing bowl, electric mixer

This fluffy buttercream is for those who view cake as the delivery vehicle for frosting. Light, airy, and yummy—you won't be able to resist licking the beaters.

12 tablespoons (1½ sticks) unsalted butter, at room temperature

2 to 3 tablespoons heavy (whipping) cream

1 teaspoon vanilla extract

¼ teaspoon sea salt

1½ cups confectioners' erythritol–monk fruit blend

1. In the large bowl, using an electric mixer on high, beat the butter, 2 tablespoons of the heavy cream, vanilla, and salt for 1 to 2 minutes, until light and fluffy. Scrape the sides of the bowl several times as you go. Add the confectioners' erythritol–monk fruit blend a little at a time. If the texture is too stiff, add the additional tablespoon of heavy cream.

2. Store leftovers in an airtight container in the refrigerator for up to 5 days.

VARIATION TIP: In a food processor or blender, grind ½ cup of freeze-dried strawberries into a powder and add it with the erythritol–monk fruit blend to make a strawberry buttercream instead.

Per serving (2 tablespoons): Calories: 83; **Total Fat:** 9g; **Total Carbohydrates:** 0g; **Net Carbs:** 0g; **Fiber:** 0g; **Protein:** 0g; **Sweetener:** 18g
Macros: Fat: 99%; **Protein:** 1%; **Carbs:** 0%

Mocha Buttercream

PREP TIME: 10 minutes
EQUIPMENT: large mixing bowl, electric mixer

This mocha buttercream will be a welcome addition to cakes, muffins, and brownies. It's light and airy with delicious chocolatey coffee flavors. What could be better than that?

1 cup (2 sticks) unsalted butter, at room temperature

2 ounces full-fat cream cheese, at room temperature

1 teaspoon vanilla extract

¼ teaspoon sea salt

2 cups confectioners' erythritol–monk fruit blend, divided

⅔ cup unsweetened natural cocoa powder, divided

1 teaspoon instant espresso powder

⅔ cup heavy (whipping) cream, divided

1. In the large bowl, using an electric mixer on high, beat the butter, cream cheese, vanilla, and salt, making sure to scrape the sides of the bowl several times. Add 1 cup of confectioners' erythritol–monk fruit blend, ⅓ cup of cocoa powder, and the instant espresso and mix until combined. Add ⅓ cup of heavy cream and beat until fully combined. Add the remaining 1 cup of confectioners' erythritol–monk fruit blend and the remaining ⅓ cup of cocoa powder and combine fully. Add the remaining ⅓ cup of heavy cream and continue mixing until fully combined.

2. Store leftovers in an airtight container in the refrigerator for up to 5 days.

VARIATION TIP: If you're not a fan of coffee or don't like caffeine, you can omit the espresso powder. You can also swap the espresso powder for instant decaf coffee powder.

Per serving (2 tablespoons): Calories: 157; Total Fat: 17g; Total Carbohydrates: 3g; Net Carbs: 2g; Fiber: 1g; Protein: 1g; Sweetener: 24g
Macros: Fat: 95%; Protein: 2%; Carbs: 3%

Chocolate Ganache

PREP TIME: 10 minutes **COOK TIME:** 10 minutes
EQUIPMENT: small microwave-safe bowl

Keep this keto-friendly chocolate ganache in your refrigerator. You'll be reaching for it often.

2 ounces unsweetened baking chocolate, coarsely chopped

4 tablespoons (½ stick) unsalted butter, melted

3 tablespoons confectioners' erythritol–monk fruit blend

¼ cup heavy (whipping) cream

2 tablespoons coconut oil

1. In the microwave-safe bowl, melt the baking chocolate in the microwave in 30-second intervals. Add the butter and confectioners' erythritol–monk fruit blend to the melted chocolate and mix until well combined. Stir in the heavy cream and coconut oil.

2. Store leftovers in an airtight container in the refrigerator for up to 5 days.

VARIATION TIP: If you don't have confectioners' erythritol–monk fruit blend, use your favorite sugar-free chocolate baking chips (such as Lily's) instead of using unsweetened baking chocolate. This allows you to omit the sweetener.

Per serving (2 tablespoons): **Calories:** 151; **Total Fat:** 15g; **Total Carbohydrates:** 2g; **Net Carbs:** 1g; **Fiber:** 1g; **Protein:** 1g; **Sweetener:** 4.5g
Macros: Fat: 91%; **Protein:** 3%; **Carbs:** 6%

Lemon Glaze

MAKES ½ CUP

PREP TIME: 10 minutes **COOK TIME:** 3 to 5 minutes
EQUIPMENT: small mixing bowl

This tangy lemon glaze is quick and easy to make and pairs well with so many different sweets. Blueberries are an especially good match.

¾ cup confectioners' erythritol–monk fruit blend

2 teaspoons grated lemon zest

3 tablespoons freshly squeezed lemon juice

2 tablespoons heavy (whipping) cream

1 teaspoon lemon extract

1. In the small bowl, combine the confectioners' erythritol–monk fruit blend, lemon zest, lemon juice, heavy cream, and lemon extract.

2. Store leftovers in an airtight container in the refrigerator for up to 5 days.

VARIATION TIP: For a lime flavor instead, use lime juice and zest in place of the lemon. You could also use orange extract instead of lemon.

Per serving (1 tablespoon): **Calories:** 14; **Total Fat:** 1g; **Total Carbohydrates:** 1g; **Net Carbs:** 1g; **Fiber:** 0g; **Protein:** 0g; **Sweetener:** 18g
Macros: Fat: 87%; **Protein:** 3%; **Carbs:** 10%

Dairy-Free Vanilla Icing

MAKES 1 CUP

PREP TIME: 5 minutes
EQUIPMENT: small mixing bowl

This icing requires just three ingredients. Easy and delicious—what's better than that?

2 cups confectioners' erythritol–monk fruit blend

6 to 8 tablespoons almond or coconut milk

1 teaspoon vanilla extract

1. In the small bowl, combine the confectioners' erythritol–monk fruit blend, 6 tablespoons of almond milk, and the vanilla. If the icing is too thick, thin with the additional 1 or 2 tablespoons of almond milk.

2. Store leftovers in an airtight container in the refrigerator for up to 5 days.

VARIATION TIP: Swap the vanilla extract for any other extract that complements the dessert you're making. For example, you could use orange extract with a pumpkin recipe or lemon extract with a blueberry recipe.

Per serving (1 tablespoon): **Calories:** 18; **Total Fat:** 2g; **Total Carbohydrates:** 0g; **Net Carbs:** 0g; **Fiber:** 0g; **Protein:** 0g; **Sweetener:** 24g
Macros: Fat: 86%; **Protein:** 4%; **Carbs:** 10%

Whipped Cream

PREP TIME: 5 minutes
EQUIPMENT: large metal mixing bowl, electric mixer

Once you've had homemade whipped cream, you can't go back to the stuff in a can. The secret of this whipped cream is the addition of cream cheese for staying power.

½ cup granulated erythritol–monk fruit blend; *less sweet: ¼ cup*

2 cups heavy (whipping) cream

1 tablespoon full-fat cream cheese, at room temperature

½ teaspoon vanilla extract

1. In the large bowl, using an electric mixer on high, beat the erythritol–monk fruit blend, heavy cream, cream cheese, and vanilla for 3 to 5 minutes, until stiff peaks form.

2. Store leftovers in an airtight container in the refrigerator for up to 2 days.

KEEP IN MIND: For best results, use a metal mixing bowl, and put the bowl and the whisk attachment from the mixer into the freezer for 10 to 15 minutes before making the whipped cream.

Per serving (¼ cup): **Calories:** 87; **Total Fat:** 9g; **Total Carbohydrates:** 1g; **Net Carbs:** 1g; **Fiber:** 0g; **Protein:** 1g; **Sweetener:** 5g
Macros: Fat: 94%; **Protein:** 3%; **Carbs:** 3%

Raspberry Sauce

PREP TIME: 10 minutes **COOK TIME:** 10 minutes, plus 20 minutes to cool
EQUIPMENT: small mixing bowl, spatula, medium saucepan, sieve

This sauce can be made with fresh or frozen raspberries. Serve it on pancakes, cake, ice cream, and more!

2 cups fresh or frozen raspberries

½ cup granulated erythritol–monk fruit
   blend; *less sweet: ¼ cup*

¼ cup water

2 tablespoons freshly squeezed
   lemon juice

1. In the saucepan, combine the raspberries, erythritol–monk fruit blend, water, and lemon juice and bring to a simmer over medium-low heat. Cook until the raspberries break apart and the sauce thickens to the point of coating the back of a spoon, about 5 minutes.

2. Pour the sauce through the sieve over the small bowl, and press through with a spatula to remove the seeds.

3. Allow the sauce to fully cool, 15 to 20 minutes, before serving.

4. Store leftovers in an airtight container in the refrigerator for up to 10 days.

KEEP IN MIND: Although straining removes most of the seeds, some will remain. This is normal.

Per serving (1 tablespoon): **Calories:** 4; **Total Fat:** 0g; **Total Carbohydrates:** 1g; **Net Carbs:** 0g; **Fiber:** 1g; **Protein:** 0g; **Sweetener:** 3g
Macros: Fat: 10%; **Protein:** 8%; **Carbs:** 82%

Brown Butter Rum Sauce

PREP TIME: 5 minutes **COOK TIME:** 10 minutes
EQUIPMENT: small saucepan

This brown butter rum sauce will add not only flavor but also moisture to your favorite cake. Perfect for bread pudding, this delicious sauce also works well on fruit or with pound cake.

6 tablespoons (¾ stick) unsalted butter, at room temperature

¾ cup plus 1 tablespoon confectioners' erythritol–monk fruit blend

⅓ cup heavy (whipping) cream

⅛ teaspoon sea salt

2 tablespoons dark rum or 1 teaspoon rum extract

1. In the saucepan, brown the butter over medium heat, stirring constantly. Once the butter begins to foam and bubble, after 2 to 4 minutes, you should begin to see browned bits on the bottom of the pan. Remove from the heat immediately and continue to stir until the butter begins to turn a golden amber color.

2. Stir in the confectioners' erythritol–monk fruit blend, heavy cream, salt, and rum until well combined.

3. Store leftovers in an airtight container in the refrigerator for up to 5 days.

KEEP IN MIND: It's best to use a stainless steel saucepan to brown butter because its light color will help you see when to take the pan off the stovetop and because it conducts heat evenly. Be sure to keep a watchful eye when browning your butter, because it can burn easily.

Per serving (1 tablespoon): Calories: 59; Total Fat: 6g; Total Carbohydrates: 1g; Net Carbs: 1g; Fiber: 1g; Protein: 1g; Sweetener: 10g
Macros: Fat: 98%; Protein: 1%; Carbs: 1%

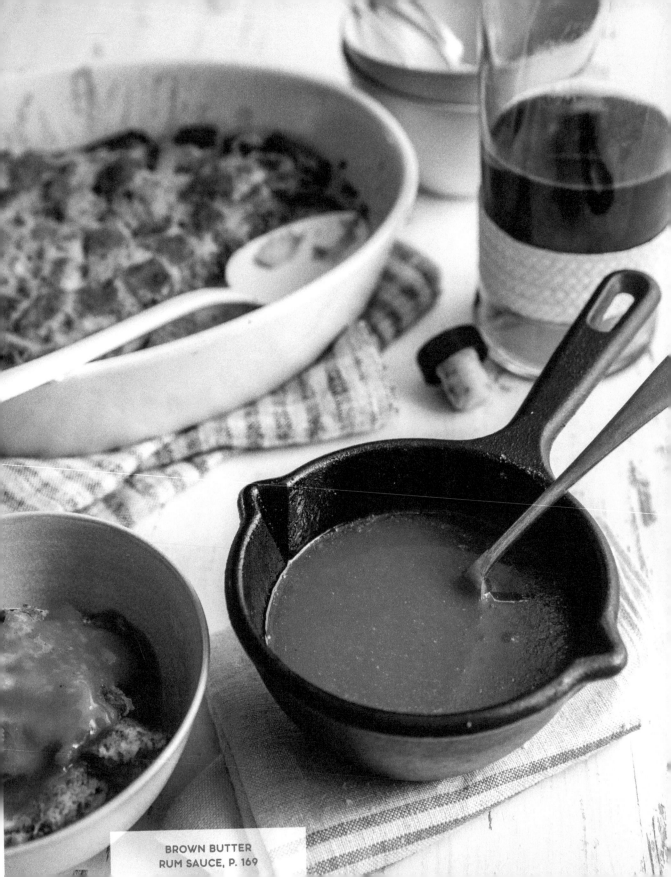

BROWN BUTTER
RUM SAUCE, P. 169

Measurement Conversions

	US STANDARD	US STANDARD (OUNCES)	METRIC (APPROXIMATE)
VOLUME EQUIVALENTS (LIQUID)	2 tablespoons	1 fl. oz.	30 mL
	¼ cup	2 fl. oz.	60 mL
	½ cup	4 fl. oz.	120 mL
	1 cup	8 fl. oz.	240 mL
	1½ cups	12 fl. oz.	355 mL
	2 cups or 1 pint	16 fl. oz.	475 mL
	4 cups or 1 quart	32 fl. oz.	1 L
	1 gallon	128 fl. oz.	4 L
VOLUME EQUIVALENTS (DRY)	⅛ teaspoon	————	0.5 mL
	¼ teaspoon	————	1 mL
	½ teaspoon	————	2 mL
	¾ teaspoon	————	4 mL
	1 teaspoon	————	5 mL
	1 tablespoon	————	15 mL
	¼ cup	————	59 mL
	⅓ cup	————	79 mL
	½ cup	————	118 mL
	⅔ cup	————	156 mL
	¾ cup	————	177 mL
	1 cup	————	235 mL
	2 cups or 1 pint	————	475 mL
	3 cups	————	700 mL
	4 cups or 1 quart	————	1 L
	½ gallon	————	2 L
	1 gallon	————	4 L
WEIGHT EQUIVALENTS	½ ounce	————	15 g
	1 ounce	————	30 g
	2 ounces	————	60 g
	4 ounces	————	115 g
	8 ounces	————	225 g
	12 ounces	————	340 g
	16 ounces or 1 pound	————	455 g

	FAHRENHEIT (F)	CELSIUS (C) (APPROXIMATE)
OVEN TEMPERATURES	250°F	120°C
	300°F	150°C
	325°F	180°C
	375°F	190°C
	400°F	200°C
	425°F	220°C
	450°F	230°C

Resources

Informational Resources

Dr. Eric Berg

DrBerg.com

YouTube.com/watch?v=vMZfyEy_jpI

Dr. Berg is one of the top ketogenic diet experts. He shares vital information on how to properly do the diet to see results. He is a health educator who specializes in weight loss through nutritional and natural methods, by combining the keto diet with intermittent fasting.

Keto Calculator

PerfectKeto.com/keto-macro-calculator

An easy, free ketogenic macro calculator that lets you add up your personal keto macros in minutes. It will help you find the exact amount of carbs, fat, and protein you need to reach your goal weight using the ketogenic diet.

Ketogenic

Ketogenic.com

A trusted resource for the keto community that offers quality education and information on the ketogenic diet. The site includes articles, tips, recipes, and tools from top thought leaders and doctors.

The Ketogenic Bible: The Authoritative Guide to Ketosis

By Dr. Jacob Wilson and Ryan Lowery, Ph.D. (Victory Belt Publishing, 2017)

This book takes a comprehensive look at the keto diet and fat-burning state of ketosis. It has the most up-to-date information on how the keto diet affects the body.

Dr. Eric Westman

Facebook.com/pages/category/Doctor/Dr-Eric-Westman-127133981830

Dr. Westman is a renowned expert in low-carb diets, diabetes and obesity, and insulin resistance. He is an associate professor of medicine at Duke University Health System and director of the Duke Lifestyle Medicine Clinic.

Online Stores

Anthony's Goods

AnthonysGoods.com
A great place to buy almond flour, coconut flour, and other alternatives to wheat flour, as well as sugar substitutes including allulose.

Bob's Red Mill

BobsRedMill.com
Bob's makes a lot of alternative flours. You can find Bob's Red Mill products in many supermarkets as well as on their website.

Lakanto Monk Fruit Sweeteners

Lakanto.com
Erythritol–monk fruit blend is my go-to choice for sweeteners. Lakanto sources all their monk fruit from the highlands of Asia, a pristine area, and using environmental methods.

OOOFlavors

OOOFlavors.com
They make delicious flavor extracts, monk fruit–based sweeteners, and sugar-free syrups.

Brick and Mortar Stores

Trader Joe's

Trader Joe's is a neighborhood grocery store with stores nationwide. It is a great place to find organic produce and products at reasonable prices.

Whole Foods Market

Whole Foods sells natural and organic foods and has a strong emphasis on sustainable agriculture. Amazon Prime Members who have stores near them get free two-hour delivery.

Index

A

Allergen substitutions, 5
Allulose, 16
Almond Chocolate Bark, 25
Almond flour, 10–11
Almond meal, 11
"Apple" Pie, 128–129
Aspartame, 17

B

Bacon Fudge, Candied, 29–30
Baking powder, 12
Baking soda, 12
Bars. *See also* Brownies
    Blondies, 75
    Blueberry Cheesecake
        Bars, 81–82
    Lemon Bars, 84–85
    Macaroon Bars, 80
    Peanut Butter Cake Bars, 83
Berries
    Blueberry Cheesecake
        Bars, 81–82
    Blueberry Crumble, 140
    Blueberry Muffins, 113–114
    Chocolate-Covered
        Strawberries, 33
    Citrus Posset, 42
    Dairy-Free Cranberry
        Muffins, 115
    Fresh Fruit Trifle, 56–57
    Fresh Strawberry Mousse, 52
    Mini Cranberry
        Cheesecakes, 103–104
    Mixed Berry Crisp, 139
    Mixed Berry Parfaits, 50–51
    No-Bake Chocolate Raspberry
        Cheesecake, 101–102
    PB and J Smoothie, 144
    Raspberry Mousse
        Tart, 132–133

Raspberry Sauce, 168
Strawberries and Cream
    Ice Pops, 155
Strawberry Mojito
    Mocktail Slushie, 149
Strawberry Rhubarb
    Cobbler, 141
Strawberry Rhubarb
    Scones, 111–112
Beverages
    Eggnog, 145
    PB and J Smoothie, 144
    Salted Hot Chocolate, 147
    Strawberry Mojito
        Mocktail Slushie, 149
Binders, 18
Blondies, 75
Blueberry Cheesecake
    Bars, 81–82
Blueberry Crumble, 140
Blueberry Muffins, 113–114
Bread Pudding, 45–48
Breads. *See also* Muffins; Scones
    Nut-Free Pumpkin Bread, 108
Brown Butter Bundt
    Cake, 88–89
Brown Butter Rum Sauce, 169
Browned butter, 21
Brownies
    Blondies, 75
    Classic Fudgy Brownies, 77
    Pumpkin Cheesecake
        Brownies, 73–74
Butter, 10, 21

C

Cakes. *See also* Cheesecakes
    Brown Butter Bundt
        Cake, 88–89
    Carrot Cake, 94–95
    Chocolate Sheet Cake, 90–91

Chocolate-Vanilla Ice
    Cream Cake, 153–154
Fresh Fruit Trifle, 56–57
Poppy Seed Pound Cake, 118
Salted Caramel
    Cupcakes, 97–98
Tiramisu, 99–100
Toasted Coconut Cake, 92–93
troubleshooting, 21
Candied Bacon Fudge, 29–30
Carbohydrates, 3–4
Carrot Cake, 94–95
Carrot Cake Cookies, 66–67
Cheesecake Fat Bombs, 35
Cheesecake Mousse, 54
Cheesecakes
    Blueberry Cheesecake
        Bars, 81–82
    Classic Cheesecake, 105–107
    Mini Cranberry
        Cheesecakes, 103–104
    No-Bake Chocolate Raspberry
        Cheesecake, 101–102
    Pumpkin Cheesecake
        Brownies, 73–74
Chocolate, 15
    Almond Chocolate Bark, 25
    Candied Bacon Fudge, 29–30
    Chocolate Chip Scones, 109
    Chocolate-Covered
        Strawberries, 33
    Chocolate-Dipped Peanut
        Butter Ice Pops, 156
    Chocolate-Drizzled Pecan
        Shortbread, 78–79
    Chocolate Ganache, 164
    Chocolate Peanut Butter
        Fat Bombs, 36
    Chocolate Peppermint
        Fudge, 31
    Chocolate Pudding, 44

Chocolate Sheet Cake, 90–91
Chocolate-Vanilla Ice
    Cream Cake, 153–154
Classic Fudgy Brownies, 77
Cookie Dough Fat Bombs, 37
Dairy-Free Chocolate
    Donuts, 116–117
Dairy-Free Chocolate
    Fudge Pops, 157
Dairy-Free Chocolate
    Truffles, 26
Dairy-Free Mocha Ice
    "Cream," 152
Dairy-Free Mocha Mousse, 53
Fudge Pie, 126–127
No-Bake Chocolate Peanut
    Butter Pie, 122–123
No-Bake Chocolate Raspberry
    Cheesecake, 101–102
Pecan Chocolate Chip
    Cookies, 65
Pumpkin Cheesecake
    Brownies, 73–74
Salted Hot Chocolate, 147
Cinnamon-Dusted Almonds, 32
Cinnamon Pecan "Apple"
    Crisp, 136–137
Citrus Posset, 42
Classic Cheesecake, 105–107
Classic Fudgy Brownies, 77
Cocoa powder, 15
Coconut
    Carrot Cake, 94–95
    Coconut Cream Pie,
        130–131
    Macaroon Bars, 80
    Toasted Coconut Cake, 92–93
Coconut cream, 13
    Coconut Cream Pie, 130–131
    Dairy-Free Chocolate
        Fudge Pops, 157
    Dairy-Free Mocha Mousse, 53
Coconut flour, 11, 14
Coconut milk
    Coconut Cream Pie, 130–131

Coconut Lime Panna
    Cotta, 49
Dairy-Free Chocolate
    Donuts, 116–117
Dairy-Free Chocolate
    Truffles, 26
Dairy-Free Mocha Ice
    "Cream," 152
PB and J Smoothie, 144
Salted Hot Chocolate, 147
Coconut oil, 10
Coffee. See also Espresso
    powder
Coffee Granitas, 150
Tiramisu, 99–100
Confectioners' sweeteners,
    16–17
Confections
    Almond Chocolate Bark, 25
    Candied Bacon Fudge,
        29–30
    Chocolate Peppermint
        Fudge, 31
    Dairy-Free Chocolate
        Truffles, 26
    French Meringues, 34
    Pralines, 27
    Salted Caramels, 24
Cookie Dough Fat Bombs, 37
Cookies. See also Bars
    Carrot Cake Cookies, 66–67
    Chocolate-Drizzled Pecan
        Shortbread, 78–79
    Iced Gingerbread
        Cookies, 63–64
    Pecan Chocolate Chip
        Cookies, 65
    Pistachio Cookies, 68–69
    Pumpkin Cookies, 70–71
    Salted Peanut Butter
        Cookies, 72
    Sugar Cookies, 60–61
    troubleshooting, 21
Cream cheese, 13
    Blondies, 75

Blueberry Cheesecake
    Bars, 81–82
Blueberry Muffins, 113–114
Bread Pudding, 45–48
Brown Butter Bundt
    Cake, 88–89
Candied Bacon Fudge, 29–30
Carrot Cake, 94–95
Carrot Cake Cookies, 66–67
Cheesecake Fat Bombs, 35
Cheesecake Mousse, 54
Chocolate-Dipped Peanut
    Butter Ice Pops, 156
Chocolate Peppermint
    Fudge, 31
Chocolate Sheet Cake, 90–91
Chocolate-Vanilla Ice
    Cream Cake, 153–154
Classic Cheesecake, 105–107
Coconut Cream Pie, 130–131
Cookie Dough Fat Bombs, 37
Cream Cheese Frosting, 160
Fresh Fruit Trifle, 56–57
Fresh Strawberry Mousse, 52
Lemon Curd Tartlets, 134–135
Mini Cranberry
    Cheesecakes, 103–104
Mocha Buttercream, 163
No-Bake Chocolate Peanut
    Butter Pie, 122–123
No-Bake Chocolate Raspberry
    Cheesecake, 101–102
Peanut Butter Cake Bars, 83
Peanut Butter Frosting, 161
Pistachio Cookies, 68–69
Poppy Seed Pound Cake, 118
Pumpkin Cheesecake
    Brownies, 73–74
Pumpkin Cookies, 70–71
Raspberry Mousse
    Tart, 132–133
Salted Caramel
    Cupcakes, 97–98
Strawberries and Cream
    Ice Pops, 155

Cream cheese (*continued*)
Tiramisu, 99–100
Whipped Cream, 167
Cream Cheese Frosting, 160
Crisps, crumbles, and cobblers
Blueberry Crumble, 140
Cinnamon Pecan "Apple"
Crisp, 136–137
Mixed Berry Crisp, 139
Strawberry Rhubarb
Cobbler, 141
Cupcakes, Salted
Caramel, 97–98
Custards
Coconut Lime Panna
Cotta, 49
Espresso Panna Cotta, 43
Flan, 40–41

D
Dairy-Free Chocolate
Donuts, 116–117
Dairy-Free Chocolate
Fudge Pops, 157
Dairy-Free Chocolate Truffles, 26
Dairy-Free Cranberry
Muffins, 115
Dairy-Free Mocha Ice
"Cream," 152
Dairy-Free Mocha Mousse, 53
Dairy-Free Vanilla Icing, 166
Dairy products, 12–13
Dairy substitutions, 5
Donuts, Dairy-Free
Chocolate, 116–117
Doughs, 4

E
Eggnog, 145
Eggs, 10
Bread Pudding, 45–48
Chocolate Pudding, 44
Classic Cheesecake, 105–107
Coconut Cream Pie, 130–131
Eggnog, 145
Flan, 40–41

French Meringues, 34
Fresh Fruit Trifle, 56–57
Fudge Pie, 126–127
Lemon Bars, 84–85
Lemon Curd Tartlets, 134–135
Macaroon Bars, 80
Mini Cranberry
Cheesecakes, 103–104
Mixed Berry Parfaits, 50–51
Poppy Seed Pound Cake, 118
Pumpkin Pie, 124–125
Raspberry Mousse
Tart, 132–133
Tiramisu, 99–100
Equipment, 18–20
Erythritol, 2, 20
Espresso powder
Dairy-Free Mocha Ice
"Cream," 152
Dairy-Free Mocha Mousse, 53
Espresso Panna Cotta, 43
Mocha Buttercream, 163
Extracts, 15

F
Fat bombs
Cheesecake Fat Bombs, 35
Chocolate Peanut Butter
Fat Bombs, 36
Cookie Dough Fat Bombs, 37
Fats, 3–4, 10, 14
Flan, 40–41
Flavoring agents, 15–16
Flaxseed meal, 11
Flours, 10–11, 14
French Meringues, 34
Fresh Fruit Trifle, 56–57
Fresh Strawberry Mousse, 52
Frostings
Cream Cheese Frosting, 160
Mocha Buttercream, 163
Peanut Butter Frosting, 161
Vanilla Buttercream, 162
Fruits, 12
Fudge Pie, 126–127

G
Ganache, Chocolate, 164
Gelatin, 18, 21
Glaze, Lemon, 165
Glucose, 3
Gluten-free flours, 4, 10–11
Granitas
Coffee Granitas, 150
Lemon-Lime Granitas, 151
Granulated sweeteners, 17

I
Ice cream
Chocolate-Vanilla Ice
Cream Cake, 153–154
Dairy-Free Mocha Ice
"Cream," 152
Iced Gingerbread
Cookies, 63–64
Ice pops
Chocolate-Dipped Peanut
Butter Ice Pops, 156
Dairy-Free Chocolate
Fudge Pops, 157
Strawberries and Cream
Ice Pops, 155
Icing, Dairy-Free Vanilla, 166

K
Ketogenic diet, 3–4
Ketones, 3
Ketosis, 3

L
Leavening agents, 12, 21
Lemons
Citrus Posset, 42
Lemon Bars, 84–85
Lemon Curd Tartlets, 134–135
Lemon Glaze, 165
Lemon-Lime Granitas, 151
Limes
Citrus Posset, 42
Coconut Lime Panna
Cotta, 49

Lemon-Lime Granitas, 151
Strawberry Mojito
    Mocktail Slushie, 149

M

Macaroon Bars, 80
Macronutrients, 3–4
Maltodextrin, 17
Mascarpone cheese, 13
    Tiramisu, 99–100
Meals, 11
Measuring, 5
Mini Cranberry Cheesecakes,
    103–104
Mixed Berry Crisp, 139
Mixed Berry Parfaits, 50–51
Mocha Buttercream, 163
Molasses
    Iced Gingerbread
        Cookies, 63–64
Mousses
    Cheesecake Mousse, 54
    Dairy-Free Mocha Mousse, 53
    Fresh Strawberry Mousse, 52
    troubleshooting, 21
Muffins
    Blueberry Muffins, 113–114
    Dairy-Free Cranberry
        Muffins, 115

N

"Natural flavors first"
    philosophy, 2
No-Bake Chocolate Peanut
    Butter Pie, 122–123
No-Bake Chocolate Raspberry
    Cheesecake, 101–102
Nondairy milks, 13
Nut flour substitutions, 5
Nut-Free Pumpkin Bread, 108
Nuts
    Almond Chocolate Bark, 25
    Candied Bacon Fudge, 29–30
    Carrot Cake, 94–95
    Carrot Cake Cookies, 66–67

Chocolate-Drizzled Pecan
    Shortbread, 78–79
Cinnamon-Dusted
    Almonds, 32
Cinnamon Pecan "Apple"
    Crisp, 136–137
Mixed Berry Parfaits, 50–51
No-Bake Chocolate Peanut
    Butter Pie, 122–123
Pecan Chocolate Chip
    Cookies, 65
Pistachio Cookies, 68–69
Pralines, 27

O

Oils, 10
Oranges
    Citrus Posset, 42

P

PB and J Smoothie, 144
Peanut butter
    Chocolate-Dipped Peanut
        Butter Ice Pops, 156
    Chocolate Peanut Butter
        Fat Bombs, 36
    No-Bake Chocolate Peanut
        Butter Pie, 122–123
    PB and J Smoothie, 144
    Peanut Butter Cake Bars, 83
    Peanut Butter Frosting, 161
    Salted Peanut Butter
        Cookies, 72
Pecan Chocolate Chip
    Cookies, 65
Pecan meal, 11
Pies. See also Tarts
    "Apple" Pie, 128–129
    Coconut Cream Pie, 130–131
    Fudge Pie, 126–127
    No-Bake Chocolate Peanut
        Butter Pie, 122–123
    Pumpkin Pie, 124–125
Pistachio Cookies, 68–69
Poppy Seed Pound Cake, 118

Pralines, 27
Proteins, 3–4
Psyllium husk powder, 18
Puddings
    Bread Pudding, 45–48
    Chocolate Pudding, 44
    Citrus Posset, 42
    Mixed Berry Parfaits, 50–51
Pumpkin puree
    Nut-Free Pumpkin
        Bread, 108
    Pumpkin Cheesecake
        Brownies, 73–74
    Pumpkin Cookies, 70–71
    Pumpkin Pie, 124–125

R

Raspberry Mousse
    Tart, 132–133
Raspberry Sauce, 168
Recipes, about, 7
Rhubarb
    Strawberry Rhubarb
        Cobbler, 141
    Strawberry Rhubarb
        Scones, 111–112

S

Salt, 16
Salted Caramel Cupcakes,
    97–98
Salted Caramels, 24
Salted Hot Chocolate, 147
Salted Peanut Butter
    Cookies, 72
Sauces
    Brown Butter Rum Sauce, 169
    Raspberry Sauce, 168
Scones
    Chocolate Chip Scones, 109
    Strawberry Rhubarb
        Scones, 111–112
Sifting, 6
Sour cream, 13
Spices, 15–16

Squash
  "Apple" Pie, 128–129
  Cinnamon Pecan "Apple"
    Crisp, 136–137
Storage, 6
Strawberries and Cream
  Ice Pops, 155
Strawberry Mojito Mocktail
  Slushie, 149
Strawberry Rhubarb
  Cobbler, 141
Strawberry Rhubarb
  Scones, 111–112
Substitutions, 5, 14

Sucralose, 17
Sugar Cookies, 60–61
Sunflower seed flour, 11
Sweeteners, 2, 14, 16–17

T

Tarts
  Lemon Curd Tartlets,
    134–135
  Raspberry Mousse
    Tart, 132–133
Tempering, 6
Thickeners, 18
Tiramisu, 99–100

Toasted Coconut Cake, 92–93
Tools, 18–20
Troubleshooting, 20–21

V

Vanilla Buttercream, 162

W

Whipped Cream, 167
Whipping, 6

X

Xanthan gum, 18
Xylitol, 17

Acknowledgments

This book is a result of years of keto dessert-making. Along the way, many people made countless contributions, both large and small, that made this project possible. I'd like to express gratitude to:

My ultra-supportive husband, Randy, who believes in me with fearless faith. Thank you for your patience, fabulous sense of humor, and for being my number one taste-tester.

Standing ovation for Michelle Gonzalez, my amazing daughter, for your incredible commitment. Without your assistance tasting, testing, and finally formatting the recipes, this book would not have been possible. You were a crucial part of this book and I would have been a complete wreck without you.

Lisa Gonzalez and Paul Molina, for being my big-hearted siblings and supporting me in every way possible, including taking care of our Mami while I worked.

Matthew Solares, my precious son who does not do the keto diet and yet willingly tasted every recipe, giving me a necessary perspective. Thanks for your honest input.

Peter, my son-in-love, thank you for your unwavering belief in me. You always inspire me to reach for the stars and take risks in the kitchen.

To my wonderful and ever-encouraging parents, Quintin and Gladys Molina, thank you. Your constant cheers always fuel me.

Thank you, Martha Avila, my mentor and beloved friend, for your faithful support and encouragement. Your example reminds me that anything is possible with the help of our Lord.

Special thanks to my pastors, Ricky and Yvette Gallinar, who believed with Randy and me when keto wasn't yet popular and supported our vision for FITTOSERVE.

Thank you to my blog followers. Your sweet tooth cravings are what propelled me to create delicious, simple keto desserts for you to enjoy.

Last, but certainly not least, special thanks to Ada Fung, my editor, and to everyone at Callisto Media who worked to make this book a reality.

About the Author

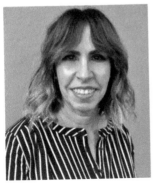

HILDA SOLARES holds a BA in theology from the Latin University of Theology. She has worked in a variety of positions in education for nearly 30 years and has more than 25 years of ministry service. In 2014, she founded Fit to Serve Group, a church community that combines the Christian faith with a low-carb keto diet. Hilda is the author of *Essential Keto Bread*, and she shares her ketogenic recipes on her blog FitToServeGroup.com through which she and her husband, Randy Solares, teach visitors to combine biblical principles with healthy eating habits for greater health and wellness. Her life's work aims to encourage people to eat well and feel well so they can serve well.